D1598742

running hot

Structure and Stress in Ambulance Work

running hot

Structure and Stress in Ambulance Work

Donald L. Metz

Abt Books / Cambridge / Massachusetts

Library of Congress Cataloging in Publication Data

Metz, Donald L.
  Running hot.

  Includes index.
  1. Ambulance service—Sociological aspects.
  2. Ambulance service—United States. I. Title.
RA995.M47   362.1'8   81-17568
ISBN 0-89011-566-4   AACR2

Printed in the United States of America.

for Mary, David, and Michael

contents

Preface

It was a pleasant Monday morning in late May when I made my first run as an emergency medical technician (EMT). Someone showed me how to check in by feeding my time card into the machine in Station 2. The crews from the first shift were rousing themselves to go home. One of the second-shift employees phoned in a request to be picked up. Amid the confusion I got the word that I would be paired with Ralph Tanner for the day. I waited for him to take the lead. He was asked, as one of the senior crew chiefs, which of the rigs he wanted, and he selected Car 33. Eventually we wandered back to the parking area to check out the ambulance.

We had just made a quick survey of the supplies in the rig and I was asking about the oxygen equipment, when Lyle came out of the back door with a slip of paper and said we had a "fire call." In company slang a fire call means an emergency run dispatched by the fire department. We jumped into the ambulance and were rolling at 8:25 AM. Tanner held the siren until we were out of the alley and turning onto the main street. Suddenly we were "running hot"—red light and siren—weaving through the early morning traffic across the city. While the rig bounced, I was struggling to get the address and type of run down on two forms and trying to keep an eye on approaching drivers. So much was happening and I was so excited that, as later became apparent, I missed most of what was going on.

The address was a run-down house divided into several apartments. It was easy to spot because the bright red rescue unit van was parked in front. On our way up to the room, the firemen pointed out that we would need a stair-chair to negotiate the narrow, twisting stairs. The patient was a forty-seven-year-old female in underpants and an open housecoat. She was unconscious but moving restlessly on the bed. Her husband said she was diabetic but that because of her condition that morning he had not been able to give her a dose of insulin. Tanner had anticipated the need and brought a tube of concentrated glucose along; he told me to try to get some into her mouth—her teeth were clamped tight—while he brought the stair-chair up. The sticky red stuff bubbled on her lips when she breathed out, but it seemed unlikely that any was getting into her system. I found it awkward to lift her into the stair-chair not only because her body was slack and heavy, but also because I wasn't used to seeing strangers in this state of undress.

We got her into the ambulance and I climbed into the back with her, alone. We headed for County Hospital. On the way Tanner called ahead to alert the hospital that we were coming in with what appeared to be a case of diabetic coma. I kept trying to get some glucose into the woman and to fill out the EMT report and the company trip slip. I tried to get a pulse but couldn't find one, although it was clear from other signs that she was alive.

The hospital staff used the empty medicine container I'd remembered to bring along to get the woman's medical records. I'd forgotten to get the husband's signature on the trip slip, I wasn't able to get a full set of vital signs, which we should have for every patient, and I hadn't done all the paperwork. It wasn't a great triumph of emergency medicine, but the patient was alive when we turned her over to the emergency department people. And I too had survived my first ambulance run. We cleared at 9:15 AM. In the next few months this would become as routine for me as it already was for Tanner. What follows in this book is a sociologist's account of how that routine develops, what it looks like, and what effect it has on the ambulance attendants and the patients.

The ambulance is one of our most visible emergency services but one of the least known. The alternating sirens, the rotating beacons, and the word "ƎƆИAⅬU𐐒MA"—ambulance spelled backward on the front of the vehicle so it can be read in a rear-view mirror—are familiar enough. But few of us know anything about the people who sit beneath the spinning lights and wailing siren or about what goes on in the back of the rig when it is "running hot."

Each year in the United States lives are lost and permanent injuries sustained needlessly because of inadequate emergency medical services (EMS). Knowledgeable people have calculated that as many as 20 percent of heart-related deaths and one-third of highway fatalities could be prevented with proper care at the scene and on the way to the hospital. Since 1970 there has been a tremendous effort to upgrade the quality and extent of these services. As a result, the United States now enjoys the best emergency medical care it has ever had. At the same time, partly because the serious development of EMS is so recent, there are numerous problems attending the delivery of this care. The problems can be seen most clearly through the eyes of ambulance personnel, who in the course of their work come into contact with all parts of the EMS system.

This study of ambulance workers is intended first of all to be a contribution to the social science literature on health care and on occupations. The book presents a sociological perspective; it emphasizes how cultural meanings, institutionalized rules, and socioeconomic backgrounds determine human activities. Though there are frequent references to individual character traits, physical limitations, and ethical dilemmas, these are not the primary focus. Of greater importance in this account are the consequences of traditional values, public knowledge, organizational authority, professional prestige, and power over resource allocations, as they conjointly limit and direct ambulance services. I try to show that many of the problems of EMS are not the result of incompetent personnel but rather are inherent in the nature of the work or are due to the way health care in this country is presently organized.

Ambulance work offers those who engage in it variety, challenge, responsibility, and above all a sense of making a valuable contribution to their community. It also offers them a lot of stress. Because this book treats their familiar world in a somewhat unfamiliar manner, I hope it will provide emergency medical personnel with a helpful analysis of the conditions that impinge on their daily work.

There is a great deal about ambulances that is dramatic, but I propose to do more than treat the subject as fascinating; I intend to treat it as important. Since most of us know little about emergency medicine until we need it, this book acquaints the wider public with how these essential activities are being handled. This report on one ambulance company is at the same time a report on the development of emergency medical services generally. It cannot but help this development to have the public know about the nature of ambulance work, its organization, its personnel, its limits.

The book begins with a discussion of the context within which ambulance work takes place. The introduction gives the reader an idea of the variety of activities, occupations, and organizations that together are called an emergency medical services system. This account is combined with a review of how historical circumstances have shaped these systems, sometimes in surprising ways. Chapter 2 describes a typical ambulance run from the time the dispatcher first notifies the crew of a distress call until the attendants signal that they are back in service and ready for another assignment. The portrayal shows all the aspects of ambulance work that are treated separately later.

The third and fourth chapters concentrate on ambulance personnel both as a group and as individuals. Chapter 3 treats the culture of the crews —the peculiarities of language and behavior that reflect the peculiarities of the work. Chapter 4 explores the routes people travel to become EMTs: where they come from, the barriers they must overcome, the nature of the training process, and the relationship between their work lives and leisure activities. It also compares this occupation with others and examines its limitations as a permanent career.

The next three chapters provide an extensive look at the interaction between ambulance personnel and their environment. In Chapter 5 we see how the employer influences the EMT's behavior both by the way work responsibilities are divided within the company and by demands that are not directly connected to patient care. Chapter 6 analyzes the contact between crews and their patients. Crews are inclined to classify their patients in terms of characteristics not associated with medical need, and these classifications affect the kind of care they offer. Chapter 7 deals with cooperation and conflict between ambulance crews and representatives of other public services, particularly fire and police personnel, and between the crews and hospitals, when they interact in the course of duty.

Chapter 8 concerns the way political actions at various levels of government affect the organization of an emergency medical services system, which in turn determines the responsibilities and future prospects of ambulance workers. The final chapter presents in conclusion a set of summary comments about the current state of ambulance services and shows how the study has implications for public policy.

A picture depends on the painter's perspective. I look at ambulance work not only as a sociologist but also as an insider (See Appendix A on participant observation). To collect information for this study, I trained and was employed as an emergency medical technician on an ambulance crew. I assumed the responsibilities and I carried home the paychecks, meager though they were. My research covered seven years, beginning with participation in an EMT course in the autumn of 1974 and ending with the preparation of this book. During that time I interviewed nearly all the EMS personnel I met; participated in two training programs; went through two sets of exams; attended dozens of council meetings, in-service workshops, and daylong seminars; clipped numberless newspapers; and regularly read a half-dozen emergency medical services publications. My employment as an ambulance attendant covered two years, including one summer of intensive work when I covered all the days of the week, both second and third shifts (I skipped the slower midnight to 8:00 AM shift). I served with all the company crew chiefs and, through occasional tours as third man, with most of the other attendants. My primary research materials were the field notes I compiled by scratching reminders on a folded sheet of paper and expanding them into full accounts as soon as I got back to my desk. These notes were supplemented by newspaper reports, magazine articles, and the few items of social science literature dealing with ambulances.

The largest part of the material came from my experience with one ambulance company. Obviously I feel we can learn a great deal from this kind of study, but we must accept its limitations. First, we must recognize that no single case is representative of all ambulance work. I know veteran ambulance workers will say certain accounts in this book do not reflect their experiences; I am equally confident they will find many similarities between their situations and the ones depicted here. It is the similarities I would like to emphasize. I have studied a private company because its personnel work full-time on the ambulances and identify themselves primarily as emergency medical technicians, rather than as firefighters or police officers. About one-quarter of the 100 largest cities in the United States rely on private companies for ambulance services. Those based in fire departments, hospitals, police departments, and volunteer organizations, as well as those considered a municipal third service, vary in particulars from the private companies. But each of them faces a set of demands and limitations that the others can recognize and appreciate. These common elements, considered in one specific context, are the chief subject of the book. Of the two main levels of ambulance work, I have concentrated on EMT-basic rather than EMT-advanced (paramedic), because basic EMTs are more numerous and less widely publicized.

Second, any account is subject to distortions because the reporter has to be selective, emphasizing some aspects and ignoring others. This study is what social scientists call ethnographic, which means among other things that I have not prettied up the picture of the ambulance worker. I have tried to be true to my experience, conveying the language as it occurred, the arguments that developed, the practices the workers actually used. It will not satisfy those readers who hold an idealized picture of the EMT; nor will it please those who consider ambulance workers to be dumbos, freaks, fakes, or failures. EMTs are ordinary people who in some ways are very special. They display a normal preoccupation with practical matters and self-interest most of the time, but occasionally they exhibit striking degrees of professional competence and human compassion.

I have tried to present actual events where possible and typical examples, except in those cases where they are noted as exceptional. However, in the interest of the analysis I have reordered occurrences and condensed conversations. Though the result is not an exact, factual account, I hope it is an accurate representation. I have used pseudonyms and fictitious details to disguise the company and the individual workers. By doing so I have felt freer to tell the truth, not because I would otherwise have exposed some serious dereliction of duty, but rather because I might have revealed some small confidence that would have unnecessarily hurt a colleague. Those who were present will recognize the participants in the story; for other readers it will make no difference.

It is the sociologist's inclination to debunk the subject of his observations, to search out and record the ways in which the practice does not match the official image. This inclination produces accounts that exaggerate conflicts, failures, and deviations. While this report will be no exception, it is subject to a balancing force. As a result of my experiences, my sentiments toward ambulance workers are largely favorable. In my opinion they are doing important work under difficult conditions with too little support. One of my intentions in this book is to present the EMT's outlook, to give a voice to those who have few opportunities to state their own case.

I am greatly indebted to the people of Liberty Ambulance Company—the owners, the office staff, the dispatchers, and especially the crews. They made the effort to educate a rookie and had the patience to put up with his questions and his strange note taking. I particularly want to thank Bill, Jim, Charlie, and J.D., who carried most of the burden. I am grateful to Linda Hall for competently and pleasantly managing the aggravating task of getting the manuscript into shape. Both the publisher and I want to thank Gary Marx, who offered encouragement and advice when they were needed and who was responsible for getting us together. The enthusiasm and guidance of the editor-in-chief of Abt Books, Bob Erwin, were valuable throughout the publishing process. I am especially grateful for the improvements suggested by my copy editor, Tori Alexander. My family has been more supportive than I deserve; Mary, my wife and colleague, should get a medal for listening to all those ambulance stories. Finally, this book is in part the payment of a debt to Harold Miller, M.D., and Evelyn Charles, R.N., who were the medical director and the instructor-coordinator of the program in which I trained as an emergency medical technician. In the face of a crowd of qualified applicants that far surpassed the capacity of the class, they decided that a sociologist might in some unknowable way contribute as much to the advancement of emergency medical services as one more registered ambulance attendant. I would like to think they made the right decision.

1

introduction

Until the early 1970s morticians operated more ambulance services in the United States than did any other kind of provider.[1] A great many seriously ill patients were being conveyed to the hospital by businessmen who often stood to gain more by the failure of their mission than by its success. The situation was illustrative of the state of emergency medical services at that time: makeshift, unregulated, ineffective.

Just as our present emergency medical services (EMS) have been shaped by the practical concerns of different branches of the health care industry, there were very practical reasons for the development of the mortician-based ambulance service, potential conflict of interest and all. Most of the funeral home providers were in rural areas where the population is thinly spread. The relatively few emergencies that would occur within the operating range of an ambulance did not justify the expense of a full-time crew. The solution was to locate someone who could provide the service as a sideline. The most obvious choice was the mortician, who was on call around the clock anyway and who had a vehicle that was suited to the transportation of patients on cots or stretchers. For the morticians it was an opportunity for community service, good public relations, and an extra return on the costs of maintaining their equipment.

The implementation of the Federal Highway Safety Act of 1966 changed the situation dramatically by setting much higher standards for training and equipment than were common in ambulance operation. Some of the funeral home providers were forced out of business. Others were happy to give it up. The latter welcomed the chance to relinquish this responsibility because, lacking adequate training, they felt uneasy dealing with critically ill persons, and because they had difficulty collecting for their services. Many morticians would have left the ambulance business sooner if they had not felt an obligation to their communities and a reluctance to leave their business rivals with what might be a competitive edge.

The responsibility for rural services has been taken up largely by volunteers, who by 1980 constituted approximately 60 percent of active ambulance personnel in this country.[2] Whether they operate as separate units or under the auspices of a volunteer fire company or a sheriff's office, these volunteers have translated emergency medical care from a profit-making venture into a public concern. Not only do they stand as symbols of the common weal by parading their equipment and their gifts of time, they force the community to share responsibility for its own medical care by requiring it to provide, usually through such joint ventures as festivals and raffles, the necessary resources. The typical citizen may even be called upon to share the inconveniences that are part of a volunteer system, as when the local barber departs to answer an emergency call in the middle of a haircut and the half-shorn customer must bide his time until a substitute arrives to finish the job. That this kind of occurrence is tolerated in a small town but nearly impossible to imagine in a city reminds us how circumstances can shape social organizations and institutions.

As for urban areas, the sponsors of ambulance services vary from one city to the next. Private companies, fire departments, police departments, sheriff's offices, city health departments, and even local hospitals serve as the auspices for emergency medical services. Which agency sponsors the services in a specific city has been decided as much by historical accident as by rational planning.

We can recognize in these few observations a summary of the current condition of EMS. First, the case of the funeral home providers shows that until very recently there was little regulation of ambulance services, and therefore there has not been time for the complete application of new standards. Second, the variety of sponsors indicates that ambulance services are neither uniform from one place to another nor coordinated by a single authority. Third, the list of sponsors suggests that many ambulances are operated by agencies whose primary purpose is something other than emergency medical services. These characteristics help to explain a great deal about the way the services are carried out today.

In order to understand ambulance work, it is necessary to know something about emergency medical services generally. And in order to get a full picture of the forces and conditions that influence emergency medical services generally, it is necessary to examine the context within which they have developed and are developing. This chapter is an examination of the context. It begins with a brief account of the historical development of the ambulance and of EMS. There follows a description of the physiological, cultural, and social conditions that have significantly affected emergency medical services. Finally, the ambulance unit itself becomes the focal point for an analysis of the social structures that provide support, operations, and control functions for it.

Historical Developments

The ancestors of the ambulance, like our own, are lost in the dim past. Understood as the transportation of the sick and injured, ambulance work can be considered to go back as far as the carrying home of the first sick child or the first backpacking of an injured companion. Even the earliest uses of devices to assist in such transportation are impossible to establish, though we know of ancient instances of the use, for example, of a hammock suspended from a single pole or from two poles (after the fashion of the modern stretcher), or of a travois in which a pair of poles is carried at one end and dragged at the other, with the patient suspended in between.

Various ingenious means of loading patients on mules, horses, and camels have been devised, and some of them have even been used. Wheeled vehicles served first as a less burdensome way of carrying hammocks and stretchers; only recently have they been designed to serve as more than mere conveyances. Streetcars, armored tanks, steamboats, helicopters, power launches, light planes, railroad trains, bicycles, and jets have all been used as ambulances.

The word "ambulance" come to us from the Latin *ambulans* (to move about) by way of a French term (*hospital ambulant*) for "itinerant hospital."[3] The Spanish army in 1487 introduced field hospitals, or special tents for the wounded, called *ambulancias*.[4] In fact warfare has been one of the prime movers in the development of emergency medical services, not only in the areas of transportation and mobile treatment facilities but especially in the improvement of triage procedures (assessment and classification of patients by immediacy of need) and emergency care techniques and equipment. The military has had both the need for such services and the opportunity to develop them.

Emergency medical care for civilians was begun before the germ theory of disease had been established and thus before the era of what we think of as modern medicine. The first ambulance service in the United States seems to have been instituted by Bellevue Hospital in New York City in 1869, though Cincinnati General (formerly Commercial Hospital) has records that show an ambulance driver on its list of employees for 1865. Bellevue intended to do more than just provide transportation; it assigned surgeons to the ambulance corps and carried first-aid equipment on board.[5] The pattern of urban hospitals providing ambulances, and of interns training by riding them, spread during the first half of the twentieth century until World War II seriously reduced the available manpower. At that point a variety of private and public organizations took over ambulance operations and created the situation in which emergency medical services were found twenty years later.

The middle of the 1960s was a watershed of sorts for emergency medical services in this country. Critics pointed out that the procedures in effect were essentially the same as those used fifty years before. Indeed, the inadequacy of the services seemed so apparent to some that they suggested emergency care be given the highest priority in our efforts to improve the nation's health.[6] A few went so far as to claim that "a dollar spent in this area would bring a greater return in the prevention of death and disability than a dollar spent in any other way."[7]

The picture that emerged as people took a closer look at emergency medical services was not a pretty one. The emergency departments of many hospitals were scarcely worthy of the name; some were not equipped as well as the minimum standards now applied to ambulances. Too often the departments were staffed by attending physicians with various specialities who took responsibility on a rotating basis and without enthusiasm. The emergency department was considered a money loser by hospital administrators. Emergency medicine was not yet recognized as a professional specialty. Ambulance services were quite diverse, but they were not closely regulated, and for the most part attendants had little training.

Perhaps the first concrete expression of recent interest in the improvement of EMS was the recommendation by the Committee on Trauma of the American College of Surgeons in 1963 that standards be established for emergency departments.[8] The Committee on Injuries of the American Academy of Orthopaedic Surgeons began in 1964 to conduct a series of concentrated courses for emergency medical personnel. In 1966 the National Academy of Sciences recognized in the title of its report on accidental death and disability that trauma was "the neglected disease of modern society."

It was the automobile and the high-speed highway that provided the impetus for change in emergency medical services. Because traffic accidents were a large part of the problem, the Department of Transportation (DOT) attempted to become part of the solution.[9] Under the National Highway Safety Act (PL 89-564) of 1966, sixteen Highway Safety Program Standards were established. Standard 11 deals with emergency medical services and requires that a certain level of emergency medical care be provided along the highway system. The act stipulates that unless states meet the standards, their federal highway funds can be curtailed.[10] However, according to its own testimony, the department was reluctant to exercise this power, a fact that some observers found discouraging.[11] DOT funding and encouragement were largely responsible for the creation of a new health professional—the emergency medical technician (EMT)—whose position indicates the minimum level of training desirable for ambulance attendants.[12] The National Highway Traffic Safety Administration (DOT) contracted to have a series of training courses for EMTs prepared.[13] Largely under the guidance of the American Academy of Orthopaedic Surgeons, the venture resulted in the development of a standard eighty-one-hour course and the publication in 1971 of a text bearing the title *Emergency Care and Transportation of the Sick and Injured*.[14]

During the late 1960s this stirring of interest led to a new sense of professional identity on the part of several concerned occupational groups. The organization in 1970 of the National Registry of Emergency Medical Technicians provided an instrument by which national standards could be employed in the certification of ambulance personnel.[15] In that same year the first residency in emergency medicine was established at the University of Cincinnati Medical Center, and a year later the Emergency Department Nurses Association was formed.[16]

While some persons were making tentative steps toward raising the quality of direct care, others were surveying existing resources to discover what conditions actually were. The findings were not encouraging.[17] By the early 1970s fewer than half of the country's ambulance attendants had been trained even to the level of an advanced Red Cross first-aid course.[18] Slightly more than one in five had been trained to the level of EMT.[19] Most ambulances were hearses, limousines, or station wagons, which did not have adequate room for proper attendant care or for storing equipment.[20] Fewer than half the ambulances could be considered properly equipped. Many lacked radio communications, particularly radio links to hospitals and physicians.[21] The staff of the emergency departments were not always well trained, and many emergency departments spent most of their time—as much as 95 percent—dealing with nonemergencies.[22] Finally, there was no uniform means by which the public could alert emergency personnel in case of a medical crisis, a situation that guaranteed a critical loss of time in taking action.[23] There were only a few notable exceptions—areas such as Jacksonville, Florida, and Seattle, Washington— where excellent EMS systems were operating.

In his state of the union message of 1972 President Nixon indicated that EMS was a national concern and should receive priority status in funding. He directed the secretary of the Department of Health, Education, and Welfare to develop new ways of encouraging and coordinating emergency medical care.[24] After opposition in the Senate and a veto by the president of an earlier version, the Emergency Medical Services Systems Act (Senate bill 2410) was passed in 1973. The main purpose of the bill was to provide incentive funds for the development of comprehensive and integrated systems for emergency medical services within geographic regions.[25] In July of 1974 the Federal Communications Commission adopted Docket No. 19880, which made several important changes to facilitate the establishment of EMS dispatch and communications systems.[26]

By 1976 advances were evident on many fronts. The General Accounting Office (GAO) surveyed developments under the 1973 act and in a report to the Congress concluded that improvement in emergency medical services "probably has caused some decreases in mortality and disability due to traumatic injury or illness," but that the regional concept of emergency care "is being compromised by virtue of the independence and differing priorities of local governments and providers."[27] The report noted that for fiscal years 1974-76 the government had put about $99 million into support of EMS programs.[28] A bill extending the EMS Systems Act of 1973 was subsequently passed; it authorized the expenditure of another $269 million on EMS through 1979.[29]

The progress noted by the GAO report was evidently based on recognized improvements in delivery of services rather than on measures of outcome for the patients. The latter are exceedingly difficult to establish; the former, though they require inferences about outcomes, are more readily obtainable. For example, the DOT estimated that by 1976 158,000 individuals had been trained as EMTs, that is, 60 percent of the 1976 category of ambulance attendants, compared with 5 percent of the 1970 roster.[30] As of July 31, 1979, 121,667 EMTs were included in the National Registry, which indicates a reasonably high standard of competence.[31] The investigators could recognize obvious improvements in equipment, since from 1966 much of the money expended on EMS by DOT was for the purchase of radios, ambulances, helicopters, and related instrumentation; more than two-thirds of the $33 million spent on EMS between 1966 and 1972 was for hardware.[32] DOT purchased about 1,400 ambulances, which was nearly one-third of the total estimated to be in operation in the United States in 1970. Improvements in the services offered by hospitals have been encouraged through a procedure called "categorization," by which, with the urging of the American Medical Association, the American Hospital Association, and several medical specialty groups, emergency departments are classified according to their relative capabilities. Equally important, the American College of Emergency Physicians by 1977 was able to list thirty-two residency programs in emergency medicine, a new specialty in the process of being recognized by the American Medical Association.

According to these and other measures, EMS has made significant advances in recent years. However, the advances have been along parallel courses rather than as a united front. Each component has been developing and improving but with much more emphasis on separate interests and activities than on their coordination. As the other side of the GAO report suggests, there are still important barriers to the implementation of efficient and effective *systems* of EMS.

The Context of Emergency Medical Services

History alone does not adequately explain the current situation. Emergency medical services, and thus ambulance units, are limited by the context within which they must operate. In some ways the context is supportive; in other respects it hinders effective action. The most important conditions affecting emergency medical services are related to human physiology, cultural values, and social location.

Physiological Conditions

Considering its complexity, the human body is enormously resistant to injury. However, if life is to be sustained, certain physiological conditions must be met. One of the most critical demands of the body is that a sufficient supply of oxygen be available to the brain. Should the supply be interrupted, in nearly all cases irreversible damage to brain cells begins within four to six minutes.[33] The destruction of brain cells in turn disrupts the regulation of essential physiological processes, such as respiration and circulation, without which normal recovery is impossible. Interruption of the supply of oxygen to the brain can be caused either by a condition that prevents the lungs from pumping air or by collapse of the circulatory system (that is, shock), so that blood no longer carries oxygen to the cells.

A second important characteristic of the human body is that nerve tissue, particularly in the brain and the spinal cord, is soft and easily injured. Any fracture or displacement of the skull or of the bones in the neck or back (or serious fractures of other bones) renders this tissue vulnerable to mutilation. Improper handling of the victims of such injuries can cause irreversible damage, which may produce extensive and permanent paralysis.

Were it not for physiological limitations such as these, an emergency medical system that emphasized speed of conveyance alone would be sufficient for our needs. However, the frequent involvement of these conditions in emergencies requires that any *effective* system include both a speedy response to calls for help and application of life-sustaining measures on site and en route to the hospital. When these measures are not taken, the well-being of the patient is threatened by every action and every minute spent in the process of loading and transporting. No amount of reckless abandon in speeding a patient to the hospital can make up for that critical time loss or for one careless movement of the injured body.

Emergency medical services have a special appeal as a means for the improvement of health care, because the application of relatively uncomplicated techniques, such as cardiopulmonary resuscitation (CPR) or the use of the spineboard, can defer death or prevent the exacerbation of injuries. Because the techniques are rather simple, they can be employed widely and at a low cost on the basis of minimal training.

The United States sustains nearly 2 million deaths each year, of which about 800,000 could be classified as medical or surgical emergencies. This classification comprises 600,000 heart attack deaths, 100,000 accidental deaths, and 100,000 deaths from miscellaneous causes. Approximately half of the accidental deaths are related to motor vehicles.[34] All age groups are represented in these statistics; while individuals over age 45 account for the majority of heart attack deaths, accidental injury is the leading cause of death for Americans under age 45.[35] In addition to these deaths, each year 2 million persons are injured in traffic accidents, and one-tenth of them suffer permanent disability. Of the 9.3 million nontraffic injuries, a quarter of a million are permanently disabling.[36]

There are good reasons to suppose that some of these deaths and the effects of some of these injuries, perhaps a significant number, could be averted were proper emergency treatment widely available. Experience has shown that the mortality rate is very high in the first hour subsequent to an acute myocardial infarction (heart attack).[37] For every thirty minutes that elapse between an accident and the administration of definitive care, the mortalilty rate triples.[38] Various interested parties have used different studies as the basis for estimates that 10 to 20 percent of prehospital heart-related deaths and one-fourth to one-third of highway fatalities could be prevented with proper care at the scene and on the way to the hospital.[39] Some of them link a sizable number of deaths and permanent disabilities directly to the actions of untrained ambulance attendants and rescue workers.[40] Finally, there is evidence that where comprehensive EMS systems are in operation mortality rates can be reduced;[41] during the first year of operation of the Illinois Emergency Medical Service System, there was an increase in the number of auto accidents and in persons sustaining injury but a *decrease* in the percentage of related deaths.[42]

Cultural Conditions

While the specific activities that shape EMS are expressed through concrete social structures, the actors themselves, both the providers and the public, are influenced by the culture in which they have been raised and by which they are sustained. Certain perceptions, or definitions of a situation, and certain values of Americans have a bearing on the status and prospects of emergency medical services. Among the more important cultural items in this regard are our attitudes toward life and death, the meaning of emergency, the assignment of responsibility for health care, and our emphasis on technology as a solution to problems.

Emergency medical services are a viable addition to the health care system because Americans value material life so highly. Such services would be of much less value in a spiritually oriented culture. If we could go so far as to say that Americans were dedicated to life at any cost, then emergency medical services would have a promising future, since they clearly save lives. However, the fact is that the American attitude toward life is ambiguous. The same people who are willing to spend large amounts of money to extend the lives of the elderly by extraordinary means also smoke, drink, overeat, and generally engage in behavior that has been shown to shorten one's life. To a large extent, it is the enjoyment of these potentially life-threatening pleasures that makes life so valuable. Americans are reluctant to pursue the latter wholeheartedly at the expense of the former.

There are not enough lives lost in emergencies to threaten a society's continuity. Therefore, measures to safeguard lives imperiled by sudden and unexpected events cannot be recommended on the grounds of societal necessity. The principal alternative is to argue that such safeguards are prudent for any individual who wants maximum protection. But the costs of emergency medical services are relatively high and are likely to require some kind of sacrifice, probably in the form of taxes, on the part of the prudent individual. Because, by the nature of emergencies, these costs are more widely felt than the benefits, the American value on life is a necessary but not sufficient impetus for the completion of an EMS system.

However much individual survival is valued and however much medical expansion is supported in that cause, emergencies constitute a category of need colored by a peculiar characteristic—they almost always happen to someone else. The experience of emergencies is not shared in the same way that we commonly suffer the discomfort of flu, near-sightedness, or low back pain. A serviceable definition describes emergency as "a situation or occurrence of a serious nature, developing suddenly and unexpectedly, and demanding immediate action." The important word here is "unexpected." Moreover, emergency is a residual category; it comprises events that fall outside the structures provided for routine, and therefore more frequent, occurrences. Both of these characteristics of emergencies, their unpredictability and their infrequency, enable us to nurture the idea that we can evade them.

Our impression that we are somewhat removed from direct involvement in the problem allows us to choose among several postures toward emergencies. The view that has probably been the most common in man's history is the one that we could call *fatalistic,* in which emergencies are considered to be an expression of fate, or the will of God, or bad luck, or retribution for past sins or carelessness, and in which it is held that since we cannot prevent these events there is no point in attempting to counter their effects.[43] The *utilitarian* variation on this view sees unattended medical emergencies as working, in the words of Dickens's Scrooge, to "decrease the surplus population," since they strike without apparent bias and effectively eliminate random members of an overcrowded society. At the opposite end of the spectrum is the *humanitarian* view, which stresses our obligation to ease the suffering of all people within our reach, including those who will be afflicted by sudden, unexpected, and serious medical problems. Finally, there is the *egocentric* view that since any individual is a potential victim of an emergency, personal security requires that the group be protected and the costs divided in order to minimize the risk of catastrophe for any one person. It is not clear that any of these views predominates in American culture, and indeed it is possible that we hold complex, even contradictory, combinations of them. The not uncommon pattern of public enthusiasm for paramedic services coupled with public reluctance to be taxed to pay for the services is perhaps nearer to the egocentric pattern than to the others.

Modern medicine has compromised the idea of emergency. Emergencies are now unexpected only with regard to the specifics of their occurrence. We know that they will occur, and statistics enable us to calculate their approximate frequency, times, and locations. Indeed, there is a class of events that might appropriately be categorized as "expected emergencies." Among others in this classification are the heart patients who carry nitroglycerine pills and a protocol to follow should an attack develop, and those who wear Medic Alert tags that describe their critical medical conditions for strangers who might attempt to give them medical assistance. Persons in this category might be expected to favor a strong emergency medical service system, because they do not share the feeling of detachment from impending threats that most of the public is able to enjoy.

Medical technology has also expanded the idea of emergency in two directions. First, by alerting the public to the potential dangers of what appear to be trivial injuries, it has encouraged people to seek immediate help for conditions that might previously have been ignored. Second, its success has convinced us that many people with conditions that not long ago would have been considered hopeless are now salvageable; where a heart attack was once interpreted as the onset of death, it is now a threatening but not necessarily fatal problem. An important consequence of this new understanding is that the public expects more from emergency care than may be appropriate. These expectations are at least in part responsible for the overutilization of emergency departments, inappropriate summoning of ambulances, and misinterpretation of the level of services available in a community. Clearly the public's definition of emergency has broadened; what is not clear is who should be responsible for delivering the necessary services and how they should be financed and controlled.

The history and organization of medicine have promoted a tremendous respect for health care professionals in this country. The public's dependence on the medical establishment is often criticized as dangerous and counterproductive for the consumer and for the society.[44]

It is understandable that this reliance on professional organizations and specialists would also characterize the public's attitude toward emergency medicine. Because few people have firsthand experience with medical emergencies, the public must base its perception of available services on fragmentary and secondary information. In part this perception is carried over from an era that produced the image of a "junior physician" leaping nimbly out of an ambulance at the accident scene, black bag in hand, ready to perfom "sidewalk surgery." In part this perception is derived from the entertainment media. Television shows, such as *Emergency,* suggest that fire companies routinely send paramedics to deal with any problem even remotely linked to health. Whatever the specifics of this perception, the public seems to assume that someone in the formal structures of government has been assigned responsibility for dealing with emergencies and that when the need arises there will be an appropriate response.

The public's assumption that there must be a reliable emergency medical response mechanism in place has at least two important consequences. First, it undercuts any popular movements to promote assessment and/or improvement of existing programs. Second, it hinders consumers from recognizing the importance of their own participation in making an emergency care system work. Bystander response is critical not only for the prompt notification of professionals, but for the aid that can be directly rendered to the victim as well. To be sure, there are reasons other than a faulty perception of available services that interfere with bystander response in medical emergencies—psychological barriers, such as "social inhibition" or "diffusion of responsibility";[45] uncertainty about legal liabilities in spite of Good Samaritan statutes;[46] and even a general cultural malaise, as in the case of the passive witnesses to the murder of Kitty Genovese. Whatever the cause of the public's reluctance to become involved, there is evidence that with proper education these barriers can be reduced. The Medic II program in Seattle has trained a sizable portion of the population in cardiopulmonary resuscitation, prompting the comment, "If you have to have a heart attack, make sure you're in Seattle."

It is important to note that significant minorities consider the public's passivity with regard to health care as worth changing. For example, some high schools have begun to teach students to monitor vital signs—pulse, respiration, temperature. In fact, the growing interest in self-care might have reached the point where it should be considered a social movement.[47] With regard to emergency care in particular, citizen groups are promoting "street medicine" as a counter to the weakness of local emergency services,[48] and instruction programs in CPR seem to be available nearly everywhere.

In short, it is important to recognize that the public's relative silence on the matter of emergency medical services is not necessarily an indication of disinterest, but could be a consequence of a somewhat distorted perception of the system already in place. There are signs that the public is willing to take a more active part in emergency care, but at present it maintains a posture of dependence on professional control, just as it does in so many areas of life.

Not only does our society seek out experts, it also is attracted to gadgets. America is aptly described as a technological culture; there is scarcely a corner of our lives that is not associated with some kind of mechanism. We are inclined to think that technological innovations or improvements are the most effective means of solving problems. In some instances our thinking is wrong, as when we shop for running gear or exercise machines as a substitute for the self-discipline that attaining good physical condition requires.

This cultural inclination toward technology is readily apparent in emergency medical services. Volunteer groups usually find it easier to raise money for purchasing a new ambulance or a radio than for operating funds or training. In its early attempts to encourage emergency medicine, the government was most concerned with purchasing equipment. Even EMS personnel display this technological bias when they recount with pride the array of pulse counters, respirators, and trauma trousers they have available.

But the value of technology is limited. It is doubtful whether even such technological cornerstones of emergency medical care as the telemetric equipment that gives the field crew the most complete consultative capacity with hospital-based specialists is useful to experienced units.[49] A bit of folk wisdom that underlies much emergency field work is that "you can do the most good by using just the equipment you get out of bed with." From this perspective, the essential elements are experienced personnel and a system for coordinating and supporting their activities. The emphasis on technology may be a popular means of avoiding the difficult task of overcoming social structural resistance to the development of coordinated emergency medical systems.

Structural Conditions

Emergency medical services, like other human activities, take place within a social structure, a network of social organizations. Just as we can describe things in terms of geographic location, we can also describe persons or jobs in terms of *social* location by indicating the groups or organizations with which they are associated, the "outsiders" with whom they have some kind of regular contact, and the agencies and officials who have authority over them. The social location of ambulance workers significantly influences how they carry out their assigned tasks.

We can understand these structural conditions most clearly by taking the ambulance unit as our central focus and noticing what affects the crew in its development and in its work. The social structures with which the crew is concerned are related to operations, support, or control functions.

Operations. Operations structures include all the people and groups with which the crew must interact while it is directly involved in carrying out its work. To begin with, it makes a difference what kind of agency sponsors the ambulance unit. Even though the training and procedures of all emergency medical technicians are pretty much alike, the auspices under which they labor affects how they do their work. For example, the public is inclined to respect the authority of an EMT in a police officer's uniform more readily than an EMT wearing the smock of a private ambulance company or even an EMT in a volunteer unit's flame-orange coverall. Or, to take another example, the possibilities for the development of teamwork depend in part on the stability of crew rosters, which in turn depends on the sponsor's personnel practices and especially on decisions about the scheduling of shifts. Regulations about the authority and duties of the separate crew members, about the availability and handling of equipment, and about records and other paperwork vary from one sponsoring organization to another and thus place different requirements on the performance of the EMTs.

The crew's operations are orchestrated by the company dispatcher, who screens calls and directs the ambulance to specific patients or scenes. The dispatcher may in turn receive assignments from a regional dispatcher, who receives all calls for emergency services in the area. Thus, the ambulance is activated by a chain of communication links rather than by direct appeal from the client-patient. Private ambulance companies may, in addition to responding to emergency calls, have arrangements with nursing homes, hospitals, and companies to transport people in medical need. The kinds of clients obviously determine to some extent how an ambulance unit manages its work.

At the scene of a medical emergency, the ambulance crew comes into contact with patients, relatives or associates of patients, bystanders, and representatives of other public services. The potential difficulty of securing cooperation from the public has already been mentioned. Not infrequently, problems of authority arise because different services with different missions are engaged in the same event. Who prevails, for example, when the EMT refuses to extricate a patient from a wrecked automobile until the fire department's heavy rescue unit cuts the seat supports, the rescue squad does not think it is necessary, and the sheriff's department wants the wreck shoved aside so it can get traffic moving again?

The final structure with which the crew is concerned in operations is the medical facility to which the patient is delivered—almost without exception the emergency department of a hospital. As a result of their repeated contacts, ambulance and hospital personnel develop personal relationships. Sometimes the associations are cordial, sometimes antagonistic. These relationships have a bearing on which hospital the ambulance attendants choose, whether they radio ahead, and how much effort they make to convey information to the hospital personnel, all of which might affect the kind of treatment the patient receives. In addition, differences in knowledge, training, or diagnosis sometimes make it difficult for hospitals and EMTs to coordinate their techniques, as when, for example, emergency department personnel want to remove traction splints or antishock trousers without taking what the EMTs consider proper precautions.

Support. The support structures are those which, though not directly involved in patient care, provide the resources used for it. In the case of the ambulance they include programs for the recruitment and training of personnel, suppliers of equipment, allied health agencies, bases of financial resources, and the approval of the public.

EMTs are usually young, male, and white. Although most of them are attracted to the work, some are forced into it—such as firefighters pressured into training because there are too few volunteers. The training programs, influenced by the Department of Transportation guidelines and directed by physicians and other health care professionals, are becoming fairly uniform. An increasing number of state and national associations promote an image of professionalism among and on behalf of EMTs and sponsor continuing education programs. However, while the standards may be set nationally, they are implemented by people associated with the local training programs. In order to insure a reasonable supply of licensees and to maintain a good teaching record, instructors are tempted to provide their students with specific hints about what will be on the examinations.

As to supplies, there are now Christmas gift catalogs of equipment for ambulance personnel, and advertising revenues in this area are sufficient to support magazines specifically for EMS workers, so that they no longer have to share the firefighters' publications. While nearly all of this equipment has a large markup, and while much of it is aimed at the vanity of the EMT who is eager to display the marks of a professional, the new interest of manufacturers has increased the availability of useful technology, such as the "trauma suits" used to control shock. At the same time, the variety of equipment in use presents a barrier to establishing equipment exchange agreements between ambulance units and hospitals.

Private health agencies are selectively enthusiastic about EMS, giving general support vocally but limiting their attention to specific aspects of the system. The Heart Association, for example, provides equipment and instructors for EMTs as part of its effort to train the public in CPR. However, the variety of interested parties within the broader area of concern occasionally leads to conflicts that inhibit systemwide cooperation. Currently, the American Red Cross and several government agencies are in disagreement about whether the backslap or the Heimlich maneuver is the preferred technique for dealing with choking.[50]

The financial support for ambulances comes from tax monies, from insurance companies, and directly from the public in contributions or in payment for services. Volunteer units have to be concerned with collecting nominal fees from users, enlisting subscribers, and running money-raising social events. Ambulances operating under the auspices of a public agency are vulnerable to budget cuts; many of them are considered by their sponsors (fire or police departments, for example) to be subsidiary services, and thus are likely to be dropped or curtailed first in a financial pinch. Private ambulance companies must invest a larger portion of their time and energy in preparing bills, insurance reports, and Medicare and Medicaid forms. Thus, the different kinds of sponsors are affected in different ways by the general economy, by policies of financial institutions, and by politics.

The stance of private insurance companies could be taken as evidence that EMS is a sound economic investment. They have testified in court on behalf of improved emergency services, and they have supported advertising campaigns to encourage people to learn CPR techniques. The assumption is that emergency care can reduce claims against the companies by limiting the extent of injuries and the likelihood of fatalities. At the same time, however, insurers use strict standards in determining whether ambulance services are necessary in an attempt to counter the public's inclination to misuse available services.

The public has been described both as insensitive to the magnitude of the problem of accidental death and injury,[51] and as a decisive force in the movement for improved medical services;[52] both as using ambulances because of manpower, speed, or official policy rather than for the skilled help aboard,[53] and as having grave misconceptions about the quality of care available.[54] The fact is that different people have different attitudes toward emergency medical services. Some portions of the public overuse emergency services,[55] while others—the more affluent—may suffer from using them too little.[56] The general public does not know much about ambulances, in many cases not even how to call for one.[57] Even those who have used ambulance services are not likely to be an effective force in their further development; they have no contact with each other, hope never to have to use one again, and thus are far from constituting a pressure group.

Control. The control structures are those organizations and agencies that do not participate in or support operations, but that do establish and enforce the regulations that control operations. Although a few regulating groups are independent, such as the National Registry of Emergency Medical Technicians, most are associated with the government. The federal government provides the impetus for applying standards to ambulances, emergency departments, EMT training programs, and others, but these standards are enforced by state and local agencies. The states, for example, usually have the final say in the licensing of ambulance attendants. The EMT is probably most aware of the local laws and ordinances that specify how lights and sirens shall be used, how fast an emergency vehicle may run, which patients must or may be conveyed, and which hospitals are to be used.

Before closing this introduction, it is important that three general characteristics of emergency medical services be emphasized. First, ambulance services are in a sense invisible to most people, because only a fraction of the population comes into contact with them. This means, among other things, that the quality of the services is not closely monitored by the public and that the public might consider support of the services a low-priority item.

Second, because emergency medical services have been so recently revised and expanded in this country, much of what ambulance personnel do has not been institutionalized.[58] That is, the culture does not yet include clear expectations about how EMTs should perform in particular situations, for example, how they should decide whether to begin CPR on a terminally ill patient. Indeed, we do not yet have standard titles by which we can refer to emergency medical personnel.[59] This book is a study of the EMT-A who has about 81 hours of training and renders Basic Life Support. The more widely known but far less numerous "paramedic" (EMT-P) has about 1,000 hours of training and provides Advanced Life Support. The public almost invariably confuses these categories.

Third, emergency medical services have for the most part been added onto already existing health care institutions—hospital emergency rooms, fire department dispatchers, private ambulance companies. The development of a *system* for coordinating these services therefore must take place within a network of habits, loyalties, and vested interests that are already associated with the necessary components. Each of the salient organizations and programs has its own idea of how such a system should work, and each is able to exercise considerable discretion within the limited sphere of its own contribution. In this situation the needs of the total system are likely to be met only after the satisfaction of what each sponsor feels to be its primary mission.

This cursory description of the context within which ambulance work takes place shows how numerous are the conditions that affect it. Each of the factors mentioned influences the way the EMT perceives, defines, evades, or accomplishes the tasks that confront him. Each leaves a mark on the central reality of the job, the activity the crews refer to as "making a run."

making a run

The Basic Unit of Ambulance Work

There are two telephones in Station 2. One is light blue, the other red. They sit at center stage in the main room of the crew quarters, sharing a table with the television set. They are of the same style, a common desktop model, and apart from color appear to a visitor to be exactly alike. Indeed, even employees, the newer ones, sometimes reach for the wrong phone. The experienced employees, however, discern a subtle difference in the bell tones of the two instruments and react differently to their signals. The red phone is usually picked up before it has rung twice and always before it has rung three times, but the blue phone may ring a half-dozen times while people banter about who should answer it.

The difference in response is due, of course, to the different functions of the phones. The light blue phone is for general use by the employees and carries all calls for them from outside the company. The red phone is reserved for calls from "base" (the Liberty Ambulance Company offices) and particularly for calls from the dispatcher. Although one of the owners, if he is also dispatching at the time, may use it to conduct routine business with an employee at Station 2, activity on the red phone almost always means a "run." A run is any assignment that involves contact with a patient or potential patient.

9:42 AM
FLASH (Picking up the red phone) *Yeah?*
DISPATCHER *I've got a call for you.*
FLASH (In mock surprise) *No shit?* (Picks up a pen tied to the desk and prepares to write on a note pad)
DISPATCHER *It's for the fire department. Eight-forty-four South Hackett Place. It's downstairs. Go in from the alley. This is for . . . squad thirty-two. Time in is nine-forty-one.*
FLASH *You got it! Say 'bye'.* (Hangs up phone. Hands note paper to Tanner, who is already putting on his jacket) *A fire call just especially for squad thirty-two. Have a good time, boys.*
TANNER (Calling to someone out of the room) *Let's go, Louie!*
Tanner and Louie leave by the back door.

The red phone controls the tempo of life in the crew quarters. It demands that someone answer it quickly. Should that person begin to take down information, the crew members scheduled to be "next out" get ready to depart even before the phone call is completed. From the first ring, momentum begins to build; from the first indication that this is a run, there is a steady movement toward the ambulance.

Rarely do the crew members tarry when they have a call, but neither do they rush. Their movements are deliberate, economical, almost a reflex action. It takes about thirty seconds from the first ring of the red phone until the duty crew is leaving the quarters. The interim is filled with certain necessary tasks—putting away (food, writing materials, model airplane kits); putting on (a smock, a jacket, an electronic pager); and collecting information about the type of run, the address, the time the call came in, and the status of the patient, if known (it usually is not).

There seem to be several reasons why the crews do not make a head-long, television-style dash for their vehicles. First, controlled haste allows a few seconds for the necessary transition from waiting to acting, a little time to break out of a TV fantasy, to wake from a nap, or simply to redirect one's attention. Second, rushing makes for mistakes—a fouled zipper, a spilled beverage, an overlooked clipboard—which may over the long haul cost more valuable time than the rushing saves. Third, the experience of crew members convinces them that there are almost no cases in which a few seconds saved on this end will make a significant difference in the out-come. Newer personnel, rehearsing in their minds the variety of disasters that might be awaiting their help, are nearly always out the door before their crew chiefs.

One other condition affects the speed of the crew's response: the type of run. Emergency runs are those that require the use of red lights and a si-ren, a procedure that is designated 10-17 in the company code. Since local emergency medical services are supervised by the fire department, these calls come almost exclusively through their dispatcher, and all calls referred by the fire department are by definition "emergencies." The larg-est proportion of the company's runs are of this type. (See Appendix B.) The second largest category comprises what are called "scheduled" runs, routine transportation of patients whose needs are known and whose transfers have been arranged in advance. A third category is known in company code as a 10-16 and includes runs in which the crew is expected to respond at once but without red lights and siren. Emergency calls elicit the swiftest response; scheduled calls, the least hurried.

9:43 AM
TANNER (Picking up the ambulance's radio microphone and thumb-ing the "talk" button) *Squad thirty-two is on the air.*
DISPATCHER *Ten-four, thirty-two. Respond ten-seventeen for the fire department to eight-forty-four South Hackett Place, apartment B. Go in from the alley. Time in is nine forty-one. K-D-J five-oh-five clear.*
In one motion Tanner hangs up the microphone and switches on the red beacons. Then he eases the ambulance into the alley behind Sta-tion 2. When they get to the main street, Louie adjusts the siren con-trol to "Yelp" and turns it on as they pull out into traffic.

At this stage of a run, plotting a route to the patient and getting through traffic safely are the primary concerns of both the driver and his partner, the "tech" (medical technician). The driver begins planning the route as soon as he hears the address. Usually the location is known to him, at least approximately, and the route simply emerges as a combination of his preferred access streets. On occasion, however, the driver is not familiar with the street or is not sure whether it connects with a particular thoroughfare. In this case the tech takes on the additional role of navigator and, using an index of street names with their coordinates and a map, plots their course while they are underway. An effective ambulance service depends more on drivers who know their territory well than on people who are skilled in high-speed driving.

The other concern, getting through traffic safely, cannot be handled so straightforwardly. An ambulance "running hot," that is, displaying red lights and siren and exceeding the normal speed limits, is quite vulnerable. For one thing, because it is designed for efficient patient handling rather than for swift running, the modern ambulance is somewhat difficult to maneuver at high speeds. Any sort of adverse weather seriously compounds this problem. However, although vehicle handling is difficult, it is at least within the crew's control and can with care be managed. The real problem, one not under the crew's control, is the behavior of other drivers.

A fast trip through traffic, siren wailing, can be as exciting to the crew inside the ambulance as bystanders imagine it to be. But there are differences. First, the personnel are preoccupied and cannot appreciate fully the thrills associated with their momentary excesses. Second, they are acutely aware of the danger of their situation and thus cannot completely enjoy the exhilaration that accompanies the risk. An attendant with even a little experience has probably had enough close calls to make him realize that avoiding accidents is something that must be worked at constantly.

Nevertheless, running hot is a form of "high" similar to that experienced by performers when they are in front of an audience. The crew is defining where the action is; faces along the way turn toward the alarming passage of the ambulance. The crew is running free, for a little while released from the rigid constraints of traffic rules, with a license to enter places from which they normally would be excluded. They are in suspense about what they will find at the scene and are aroused by the urgency implied in every part of their routine. All these feelings are heightened by the fear that comes and goes as other vehicles threaten to collide with them and then are left behind. The crew's world shrinks until it consists of little more than the ambulance and its immediate environment.

Running hot is the most intense time in ambulance work. The driver is engrossed in maneuvering the rig, watching the traffic, and staying on the route. The tech is "driving the right side" (watching for traffic coming from the right at cross-streets where a traffic signal or stop sign is violated), working the siren, watching the street signs and house numbers, and begining to record information about the run on standard report forms.

These are the routine assignments of the crew. In addition there may be problems with the route that require extra navigation or radio conversations that both relay additional information and distract the crew.

9:44 AM
DISPATCHER *Dispatch to squad thirty-two.*
TANNER (Grabbing the microphone with his right hand) *Thirty-two. Go.*
DISPATCHER *The rescue unit on the scene says you'll need oxygen.*
TANNER *Ten-four.* (Hangs up the microphone)

These activities take place while street scenes are flashing by the windows, the rig is bucketing and bouncing over rough pavement, and the cab is filled with the piercing noise of the siren. Incredibly, the crew has time to attend briefly to matters unrelated to the run:

9:45 AM
TANNER (Shouting over the siren as he begins to slow for the turn onto Spring Street) *There's the Ardmore! That's the place I was telling you about!*
LOUIE (Switching the siren from "wail" to "yelp" as they catch up to a clot of cars) *Yeah, I remember!*

The tech, driving the right side, shouts (to be heard over the siren) "clear" or "clear right" when he is as sure as he can be that nothing is entering the intersection from that direction. Because many intersections are "blind" and cannot be adequately scanned from a distance, and because the average driver's intentions are sometimes obscure, even if he can be seen, running hot is at best a slow-and-go operation. Obviously, the fewer the occasions on which one has to slow down, the faster the running time. For this reason, drivers choose their routes largely to avoid stop signs, particularly those at blind or busy intersections. Another important consideration is whether the traffic signals on the street are "timeable." An experienced driver will know that at a steady speed of 48 miles per hour it is possible to catch every traffic light green on a particular downtown street that has a posted speed limit of 30 mph. From the driver's point of view, this course of action is safer and more efficient than the company's policy that ambulances should stay within 5 mph of the posted speed limit.

The main means of alerting the public to the presence of an ambulance is the siren, supplemented on rare occasions by the air-horn or the loudspeaker. The most familiar siren in America is the "wail," which is a slow modulation from low to high frequency and back; it is used on relatively straight and uncongested stretches. At intersections or where traffic is dense, the crew will usually switch to the "yelp," a rapid modulation between the same frequencies. It seems to convey a greater sense of urgency, as well as providing a better basis for discerning the direction of the ambulance. The "two-tone" or "high-low" is a steady alternation of two frequencies. It is widely used in Europe but is less common in this country, though its unfamiliarity makes it useful at times, particularly when there is a danger that the conventional sirens of two emergency vehicles known to be approaching the same location might mask each other.

Unfortunately, the effect of the siren has been seriously compromised. For one thing, sirens are so commonplace in cities that even pedestrians scarcely look up these days to note the passing of an emergency vehicle. For another, the urban setting neutralizes much of the effect of the siren. Sounds in a downtown area ricochet off building walls like echoes in a river canyon, making it difficult, and perhaps impossible, to locate an emergency vehicle precisely. Even flashing red beacons are inconspicuous against the background of display, street, and vehicle lights on and along city streets. Finally, as automobiles have become more luxurious, they have more effectively screened their drivers from the influence of the environment. With the windows closed, an air conditioner or heater working, and a radio or tape deck playing, it is unlikely that a driver will be aware of the approach, always unanticipated, of an emergency vehicle. These circumstances produce a problematic situation in which pedestrians complain that they can't stand the sirens, and drivers complain that they can't hear them.

The safe passage of an ambulance is not assured even if the siren attracts the attention of other drivers. Frequently traffic reacts to a siren like the inhabitants of a disturbed anthill, scattering in all directions. The correct procedure in most states is for traffic to move as far to the right as possible and to remain there until the emergency vehicle has passed. Often, however, people simply stop in the middle of the roadway. The ambulance driver can never be sure whether a particular automobile will remain stationary or perhaps, in an attempt to get out of the way, suddenly swerve into the path of the rig. In the final analysis, the crew's best protection is defensive driving—assume other drivers will make the worst possible decisions and be ready at all times to take evasive action.

9:47 AM
LOUIE (Shouting as they pass an intersection) *That's Columbia! Hackett's next! We want the alley on the far side!* **(Kills the siren as they start the turn into the alley. Ahead they see the rescue unit's parked rig with the red beacon turning on top)**
TANNER (Picks up the microphone) *Squad thirty-two is ten-twenty-three.*

DISPATCHER *Ten-four, thirty-two.*
Tanner replaces the microphone and parks the ambulance. Louie
records the time of arrival on the scene. As they climb out, a member
of the fire department's rescue unit approaches them.
FIRST FIREFIGHTER *You'd better bring your oxygen. She seems to*
be having some trouble breathing so we've got her on oh-two. (Walks
with them to the back of the rig, where they get out the wheeled cot
and load it with the green oxygen tank, a nose piece for the oxygen,
and the clipboard)
This is a woman who passed out sometime this morning but wasn't
discovered until about a half-hour ago. She's still out. We got some
vitals. A friend from upstairs is with her but she speaks Spanish and
we can't get much information. May be a drug overdose.

The crew members anticipate the characteristics of a run in very general
terms. They are concerned about what kind of equipment they might
need, the kind of building they might encounter, the kind of people they
will have to deal with, but there is no way they can prepare for the specific
medical problem they will face. The ambulance responds to most of its
calls with minimum information: time, location, and type of run. Scheduled calls almost always include details about the patient's condition; emergency calls almost never do. Moreover, there is a good chance that when
details do accompany an emergency call, they will be inaccurate due to the
panic and inattention of the caller and the haste and preoccupation of the
dispatcher. A call presented to the crew as "female, pregnant, with contractions three minutes apart" (and thus apparently ready to deliver
momentarily) may in reality be a woman with a bellyache who has not
even noted the regularity of her pains, let alone timed them. Experienced
EMTs seem to agree that it is pointless to worry about the specifics of the
case until you are on the scene.

Nevertheless, the crews do try to predict the kinds of cases they will find
by using the time and location as the basis for their estimates. Particular
kinds of emergency calls are associated with particular times of the day.
Industrial accidents are naturally more frequent during working hours; traffic accidents occur during (commuter) "drive time" and in the early evening; drunks and fights are more prevalent in the hours of darkness. Location is also an informative clue to the nature of the call. For example, traffic
accidents will be described by the dispatcher in terms of cross-streets or
freeway exit ramps. Through experience the crews learn the addresses of
certain notorious bars, of the flophouses and rescue missions, of the jails,
of apartment buildings that cater to the aged, and of certain "regulars" who
frequently ask for ambulance services. In addition, the crews categorize
sectors of their service areas in terms of the clientele most often encoun-

tered there—Little Puerto Rico (Hispanics), State Street (skid row bums), The Industrial Valley (blue-collar workers), The Lower East Side (hippies and junkies), and so on. The presumed nature of the call affects at least the degree of enthusiasm with which a crew pursues its mission. Personnel eagerly depart for a traffic accident, which is considered a "good" run, but tend to linger if bound for the Rescue Mission to "haul a drunk,"

9:48 AM
The crew maneuvers the cot into Apartment B. A woman in early middle age is lying on the sofa tossing restlessly. A pale green oxygen mask covers her lower face. A firefighter is kneeling beside the sofa trying to time her breathing. Another woman and another firefighter are talking in the kitchen area. A cluster of people, including a few giggling children, look in through the open front door.
SECOND FIREFIGHTER (Looks up from where he is kneeling) *Her B.P. is a little low. Here are the vitals.* (Hands a paper to Louie, who has begun to fill out a form on the clipboard) *We got her name from her friend there, but that's about all. She found her like this about twenty minutes ago. Doesn't smell like booze.*
TANNER (Adjusting the cot so the bed is about level with the sofa seat) *Find any medications?*
SECOND FIREFIGHTER *Yeah. This was on the table there.* (Hands Charlie a plastic container with several pills in it) *No label. The other lady doesn't know if she was taking anything. Or she won't say. I'll give you a hand.*
Tanner and the second firefighter lift the supine body onto the ambulance cot. Louie tries to ask the patient's neighbor if she will accompany them to the hospital. She vigorously shakes her head in the negative. Louie slips the clipboard under the pillow on the cot and helps to wheel the patient through the door.
TANNER (To the first firefighter) *We'll take her to St. Christopher's. Will you close up here?*

At the scene there is always more confusion than anyone expects. The curiosity of bystanders alone helps to transform an occasion for the simplest procedures into what looks like a major crisis. By the time family members and representatives of two or more service groups (police, fire, ambulance) have crowded into a room with the patient, there's considerable commotion. The crowd's excitement, the anxiety and embarrassment of family or friends, and the multiple purposes and intrusive manner of service personnel make it difficult to discover and sustain a shared definition of the situation.

The purposes of the ambulance crew at this stage are two: to assess the patient's condition and to stabilize the patient for transportation to the hospital. The assessment, or initial patient survey, is intended to identify those emotional and physical problems which, if unnoted, will result in death or serious deterioration of the patient's condition.[1] In theory it is a hands-on, four-senses (taste is excluded), head-to-toe physical examination,[2] combined with the collection of all information relevant to the present condition of the patient. In practice the EMT usually makes sure the patient's breathing and circulation are adequate, then concentrates on the primary complaint. For example, an elderly patient who complains of shortness of breath, but who has not suffered any physical injury recently, is not likely to be carefully checked for possible broken bones.

The "primary complaint" is defined by the patient and/or the family and is the expressed reason for summoning the ambulance. From a physician's point of view, it may be of secondary importance to another condition that receives little attention. For example, a patient may black out for a moment and fall; when the ambulance is called, the primary complaint is a relatively minor injury sustained in the fall, though the condition that caused the loss of consciousness is a much more serious problem. Frequently the primary complaint is not self-evident but rather a general feeling that "something's not right" or a combination of several ailments. Whether there is an apparent ambiguity or not, the crew must make a conscious effort to clarify the primary complaint as much as possible.

Three sources of information are available to the crew. The patient is probably the most knowledgeable informant about the case, but an unconscious, semiconscious, or severely distressed patient cannot provide the necessary information. The next most important informants are the close family and friends of the patient, but their accounts are almost inevitably inconsistent, garbled, or fragmentary. In those rare moments when people are closely questioned, it becomes uncomfortably clear how little they really know about the habits, feelings, and condition of those with whom they are intimately associated. Language differences may further reduce the meager store of information that can be gathered from these associates. Finally, physical clues can help explain a patient's condition; residues of vomitus and blood, drug containers, personal documents, and especially diagnostic signs—pulse, blood pressure, respirations—usually are considered the most reliable evidence on which conclusions can be based.

The ambulance crew does not have a free hand in assembling a set of accurate facts on the patient's condition. In many cases the information it receives is screened by the "first responders," the service personnel (usually police or firefighters) who arrive earliest on the scene. For example, where the fire department is responsible for EMS, the firefighters will respond to a call first, make a rapid estimate of the need for further help, and, once they have called for an ambulance, continue to collect information from the family while they await its arrival. Because of social pressure resulting from this procedure, the ambulance crew is to a very large extent dependent upon the first responders for their information. At the least it is somewhat awkward for the crew to ask the family, in whose eyes speed is of the essence, to go over the same ground that has just been covered by the first responders.[3] Beyond that it might be considered an impugning of the first responder's skill if the ambulance crews want to go to the original sources rather than accept someone else's version of the facts. The degree of constraint in questioning that the crew feels varies according to specific conditions and the personal relationships with the individuals involved. A desire to avoid upsetting the family or alienating the first responders inclines the crew to accept information that has been edited.

The disadvantage of this screening is that the first responders might, in spite of their best intentions, alter the characteristics of the case. The most obvious distortions result from ignoring or forgetting information (the patient had been hospitalized briefly last month) and from getting facts confused (reporting that the patient began to have a seizure and then fell, rather than the reverse). Forgetting and ignoring are often signs of a more subtle and influential cause—the tendency to make a diagnosis and then select perceptions to support it. This tendency is characteristic of many kinds of investigators: "Basically, they all use the *a priori* method. . . . The policeman will always construct an initial view of things, sometimes within a few seconds of arriving on the scene, and the evidence, as it filters through to him, will be made to conform."[4] No one is immune to this tendency, and the patient is subjected to a kind of double jeopardy when the ambulance personnel are pressured into adopting a second-hand interpretation of the situation. The first responders typically greet the crew with a plausible explanation of the patient's problem. While the crew members are not bound to accept this diagnosis, they cannot escape being influenced by it, both because it provides a ready answer to the question that is uppermost in their minds at the time and because it has shaped the information that is passed on to them.

The ambulance crew does not naively accept the first responder's depiction of the patient's condition, however. Ambulance personnel frequently express cynicism about the medical ability of the personnel of other services, in part at least because of the competitive tension between different groups engaged in similar work. The skepticism is evident in efforts to protect themselves from the possibly faulty diagnoses of their collaborators. EMS reports are carefully annotated to indicate that a particular evaluation was "according to" the first responder or that the first responders had applied a bandage or air splint that was not removed or altered by the ambulance crew. Thus, the crew members may utilize the first responder's definition of the medical situation, but they are aware of what they are doing and are cautious about it.

The ambulance crew's second responsibility at this point is to stabilize the patient for transportation. In practical terms this means taking precautions to insure that the patient's condition upon leaving the ambulance is no worse than when first entering it. It involves the initial treatment of potentially serious problems, such as hemorrhage or fractures, and the anticipation and prevention of life-threatening conditions, for example, shock—the collapse of the circulatory system. The current rationale of EMS is that a few minutes spent at the scene making sure that the patient's difficulties will not be exacerbated during the trip eliminates the need for running hot to the hospital, thus reducing the level of danger to the patient, the crew, and the public.

9:59 AM
Tanner and Louie lift the cot into the back of the ambulance and lock it to the sidebar. Louie gets in and switches the oxygen line from the portable tank to the stationary supply. Tanner closes the back doors and goes around the outside of the rig, climbs into the driver's seat, fastens his seat belt, and starts the engine.
TANNER (Picking up the microphone) *Thirty-two to dispatch. We are en route to Christopher's with one.*
DISPATCHER *Ten-four, thirty-two.*
TANNER (Leaning over to look back through the access port into the rear compartment) *You want to get a blood pressure before we move out?*
LOUIE (Already attaching the blood pressure cuff to the patient's arm) *Yeah, give me a minute.* **(Inflates the cuff and watches the dial on the action wall while he listens through the stethoscope for a pulse)** *Okay.* **(Takes the stethoscope off and begins to fill out the EMS report while the rig pulls out of the alley)**

The physical condition and the personality of the patient determine what happens in the back of the ambulance on the way to the hospital. The first responsibility of the tech who is riding in back is to monitor the patient's state of health. The most extreme cases, and thus the most infrequent, are those in which the patient's condition is deteriorating so fast that the ambulance must run hot to the hospital. The most extreme case of all is the patient who "codes" while en route. That designation is taken from the practice in hospitals of announcing a "code blue" or "code four" to summon staff when a patient suffers a respiratory or cardiac arrest. When a patient becomes a "pulseless nonbreather" in the back of an ambulance, the tech lets the driver know—"Haul ass, Charlie, we've got a code"—and immediately begins CPR (cardiopulmonary resuscitation, the term for mouth-to-mouth ventilations and chest compressions), which he continues until the emergency room staff takes over or the patient revives.

In serious cases the tech's monitoring involves a regular checking of vital signs—respirations, pulse, blood pressure. In most cases the patient is conscious and much of the monitoring can be done by questioning along with observations of complexion and body movements. The tech's evaluations of patients are influenced to some extent by his recognition that people are not uniform in their reactions to pain—some are frantic about minor discomforts while others give little indication of the agony associated with major injuries.[5] Because these reactions vary from individual to individual, the tech's scanty knowledge of the patient provides no basis for making fine distinctions. Instead he is forced to make his assessment on the basis of sweeping generalizations derived from his experience and from the crew culture. In practical terms, the tech develops broad characterizations of the typical behavior of categories of patients—women are more emotional about injuries than men, the well-to-do elderly complain more than the poor elderly, and so forth—and adjusts his interpretation of the patient's behavior in terms of these generalizations. Probably the tech is more likely to underestimate the misery of emotionally demonstrative patients than to overestimate the distress of quiet ones, in large part because the unmanageability of the former is irksome. Techs will, though rarely, talk harshly to patients whose lamentations they consider excessive. If the patient is both talkative and self-controlled, the tech's work is easier in that he can do much of his monitoring with his ears.

While conscious patients may be easier to monitor, they also require more reassurance. Techs work out ways of quickly conveying to them a sense of the supportive attitude expected of ambulance personnel. The techniques include periodically asking how the patient feels, establishing physical contact by feeling the forehead for temperature or taking a pulse, commenting on the route the ambulance is taking, and even fashioning conversational routines designed to lighten the atmosphere—"Yeah, it is a little bumpy back here. I hear this is pretty close to what it feels like to ride a three-legged camel." Providing reassurance can become a trying business for the tech if, for example, the patient is both anxious and deaf, or the patient uses this opportunity to complain about an apparently endless list of grievances.

10:03 AM
TANNER (Calling through the access port) *Are you ready to talk to St. Christopher's?*
LOUIE *Yeah, I'm ready.*

TANNER (Thumbing the button on the mike) *Thirty-two to dispatch.*
DISPATCHER *Go ahead, thirty-two.*
TANNER *We're going to frequency two.*
DISPATCHER *Ten-four, thirty-two.*
Tanner punches out a three-digit hospital code on the encoder.
RADIO VOICE *St. Christopher's emergency department.*
LOUIE (Taking the phone handset from the action wall) *St. Christopher, this is Liberty Ambulance Squad thirty-two. We are en route to you with a female, approximately thirty-five years old. Semiconscious. Cause of problem unknown. Possibly drug-related. Her BP is one hundred over sixty-five. Pulse: ninety and strong. Respirations: twenty and shallow. Our ETA is three minutes from now.*
RADIO VOICE *Thank you, Liberty. KLM 23185 clear.*
LOUIE (Hanging up the handset) *Okay, Tanner.*
TANNER (Adjusting the radio and picking up the mike) *Thirty-two is back on frequency one.*
DISPATCHER *Ten-four, thirty-two.*

The second responsibility of the tech in back is to handle the paperwork. A form widely used by ambulance units is the standard EMS report (see Figure 1), which includes data on the patient, a checklist account of the patient's condition, a record of the treatment given in the ambulance, and a brief description of the nature of the specific problem. In addition, private companies use a "trip slip" on which the EMTs enter information pertinent to billing the patient for costs and on which the patient's signature is required. Public service organizations have their own systems for logging information on the runs made by their units. One of the most useful skills an EMT can have is the ability to write legibly in the back of a moving ambulance. As often as they can, techs use the question-and-answer work required by the reports as part of their monitoring.

10:08 AM
The ambulance slows to make the turn into the drive marked by a large red arrow inscribed with the word "Emergency,"
TANNER (Picking up the mike) *Thirty-two is ten-twenty-three St. Christopher's.*
DISPATCHER . . . *Four, thirty-two.*
Louie disconnects the blood pressure cuff and moves the oxygen line to the portable tank. Tanner comes around the outside and opens the rear doors. Louie gets out and they lift the cot down and readjust the bed to waist height. As they begin wheeling it toward the doors marked "Emergency Entrance," a young woman with a clipboard comes out of the emergency department admitting office and begins to question them about the patient.

Figure 1
EMS REPORT FORM

SERVICE: _____ ID # _____ No. _____ Date _____ Mo. Day Yr.

Station _____ Ambulance # _____	Run/ Alarm # _____	TYPE OF DISPATCH: ☐Non-Emer. ☐Standby ☐Emergency ☐Emer. Transfer ☐Drill

Pt. Detected _____
Call Rec. _____
En Route _____
At Scene _____

LOC. OF PICKUP _____

ATTENDANTS		CIRCLE	Lv. Scene _____
EMT in charge	1. _____ 2. _____ 3. _____ 4. _____	A.M. P.M.	At Dest. _____ In Service _____ (Use Military times)

TWP/City _____ (County)

CALL REQUESTED BY: _____ MILEAGE: End _____

PATIENT NAME _____ PERSONAL PHYSICIAN _____ Begin _____ Total _____

ADDRESS _____ MEDICATIONS WITH PATIENT _____ PATIENT ZIP CODE

☐Airway Obstr.	☐Airway Cleared	☐Airway Inserted	☐Endotracheal Tube	☐Oxygen ___L.	☐Suction Used	☐Respiratory Arrest
☐Acute Cardiac	☐Arrest	☐Chest Pain	☐Defibrillate	☐ ___ w/s	Time CPR Started _____ Time CPR Stopped _____	
TRAUMA ☐Major ☐Minor	☐Spinal Col. Inj.	☐Long Backbd ☐Short Backbd	☐Cerv. Col. ☐Head Inj.	☐Fractures ☐Traction ☐Splints-kind _____	☐Bleeding ☐Bandage	

OTHER MEDICAL PROBLEMS:
☐Shock ☐Exposure
☐Stroke ☐Alcohol
☐Acute Psychiatric ☐Drug
☐Poison _____ (agent)
☐OB-GYN ☐C.B. ☐Miscar.
☐Other Illness _____

CAUSE OF INJURY: ▶

MENTAL STATE:	CHECK ALL THAT APPLY	TRAUMA (ENTER NUMBERS OR DRAW LINES)
INITIAL STATE: ☐Alert ☐Semi-Con. ☐Uncon. ☐Prob. Dead	☐Normal ☐Confused ☐Sleepy ☐Slurred Speech ☐Abnormal Behavior ☐Unresponsive	☐Pt. Reassured ☐Intermittant Consciousness ☐Incoherent ☐Verbal ☐Pain Stimulus

1. Fracture
2. Dislocation
3. Pain
4. Bruise
5. Laceration
6. Avulsion
7. Burn
8. Abrasion
9. _____

SITES

SYMPTOMS	EYES	SKIN	INITIAL FIRST AID:	Who? What?
☐Vomit/Naus ☐Convulsing ☐Combative ☐Fever ☐Cold ☐Dizziness ☐Numb/paral.	R Normal L R Constricted L R Dilated L R Nonreactive L	☐Normal ☐Moist ☐Cold ☐Flushed ☐Pale	_____ _____ _____	

SEX M F   DOB or AGE

MEDICAL HISTORY		
☐Heart Disease ☐Diabetes	☐Epilepsy ☐Psychiatric ☐Other	☐Med. ID _____ ☐Allergy _____

IF JOINT INJURY CIRCLE INJURED AREA ON FIGURE.

TIME	B/P	Pulse		Resp.		EKG	Medication			Consciousness				Pupils	Gen. Cond./
		Rate	Qual	Rate	Qual		Drug	Dose	Route	No Chg	More	Less	UNC.	Size Change	Treatment
			Reg IRR.		LAB SHALL CH/ST.							/		R UNCH. L R INCR. L R DECR. L	

COMMENTS/OTHER TREATMENT

URGENCY:	☐Life Threatening	☐Acute, Non-Life Threatening	☐Non-Emergency	☐Run Cancelled (Why) _____	
ACTION:	☐Transport and Care	☐At Scene Care Only	☐Exam Only	☐Patient Refused Exam	
NO TRANSPORT:	☐No Patient	☐No Need	☐Patient Refused	☐Went By Other Means	☐Release Signed
TRANSPORTED ON:	☐Back	☐Side ☐Stomach ☐Sitting	☐Other ☐Head Elevated	☐Feet Elevated	☐Restrained
DESTINATION:	☐Hospital	☐Nursing Home ☐Other	REASON: ☐Patient ☐Physician	☐Closest ☐EMT Choice	
WHERE:			☐Medical Need	# I.V. Attempts: _____ Successful? Y___ N ___	
ARRIVAL STATUS:	☐Unchanged ☐Better ☐Worse	☐D.O.A.		Where? _____	
PT. ADMITTED:	☐E.D. ☐CCU ☐ICU ☐Other	E.D. #		E. D. Physician: _____	
CONTACT WITH HOSPITAL	☐Radio ☐Phone ☐Direct ☐EKG Telemetry			Time Report Received: _____ By: _____	

AMBULANCE REPORT SYSTEM, BUREAU OF HEALTH STATISTICS, BOX 309, MADISON, WI 53701

HOSPITAL COPY

There are still a few hospitals with emergency rooms that are less well equipped than the ambulance that delivers patients to them. In these places it may be difficult to find someone to take responsibility for a patient. However, these days one is likely to find so many staff members hanging around the emergency department (ED) it is hard to tell who is in charge. This is especially common in the large hospitals frequented by city ambulance services, and it occasionally presents a problem for the crews. They are interested in transferring information along with the patient, but it is sometimes difficult to find someone who is interested in receiving it. Inside the doors of the ED there is likely to be a crowd of people in uniforms, all with stethoscopes around their necks and with name tags too small to be read from across the room. The tech wants to make a report to a responsible party but cannot tell the doctors, aides, nurses, and orderlies apart.

The solution to this problem is usually experience. Over time the EMTs learn who are the people in charge in the various EDs and thus know after a while to whom to report. The ED personnel begin to make evaluations of the EMTs and form an idea of which ones are worth listening to. The staff members are inclined to trust only the information they gather from their own observations and to mistrust the reports of outsiders, much as the ambulance crews mistrust the diagnoses of the first responders. In cases with no striking peculiarities, the report of the EMT is little heeded. Nevertheless, the EMT does not consider his work finished until he has made a report, and he may in desperation speak to anyone who will listen.

10:10 AM
LOUIE (To nurse who approaches them) *This is the possible O.D. we called about.*
HEAD NURSE *Okay. Let's see . . . six is empty.* (To another nurse) *Chris, put this one in six.*
TANNER (Hands the head nurse the pill container) *These were in the room with her.* (Louie wheels the cot to the cubicle)
DR. CATALDO (Watching from behind the desk at the nursing station) *May I see those, please?* (Empties the pills into her hand) *Could be street drugs. I don't know.* (Replaces the pills and hands the container to an orderly who has just walked up) *See if the pharmacy can tell us anything about these.*
Tanner, who has been looking on, moves off toward the cubicle to help shift the patient onto the bed.

Once the patient has become the responsibility of the hospital staff, the urgency diminishes for the ambulance personnel. They must complete the paperwork about the run, collect signatures where necessary and possible, replace certain expendable equipment from hospital stores, and clean up. Though the emergency character of the run has disappeared. the EMTs will often hang around for a while out of normal curiosity and professional interest. They would like to know the official diagnosis of the problem, how the patient is handled, and what they might have done to improve their own performance, though they can rarely stay around long enough to hear about the definitive treatment of an ambiguous case. For many of the crews, lingering has the added attraction of making it possible to flirt with some of the hospital staff. It is not unusual for acquaintances struck up in this way to lead to leisure time relationships and occasionally even marriage.

10:22 AM
Tanner and Louie are at the back of the rig putting a clean paper sheet on the cot, following a routine they have been through together many times. They refold the blanket and towel and stow a clean sheet and a new absorbent pad under the pillow, then close the cot straps over the pillow and blanket. In unison they lift the cot and lock it in the back of the ambulance. Louie climbs into the back and refolds the blood pressure cuff; Tanner goes around the outside and gets into the driver's seat. After climbing through the access port to the passenger's side of the cab, Louie staples the EMS report and the trip slip together and drops them into a file box. He sets up the next set of reports as Tanner backs the rig out of the ED parking area.
TANNER (Keying the mike) *Thirty-two to dispatch.*
DISPATCHER *Go ahead, thirty-two.*
TANNER *We're ten-twenty-four and ten-eight at St. Christopher's.*
DISPATCHER *Ten-four, thirty-two, you're ten-nineteen.*

Radio conversation is kept to a minimum both as a matter of company policy and because of government regulations. The EMS bands are restricted to business communications and are known to be monitored by the regulating agencies. Consequently, there is little chatter on the radios, and attendants will occasionally discuss whether a particular dialogue ("Squad Thirty-two, would you please give me your odometer reading?") is a legitimate use of the radio or should have been handled by land line, that is, by telephone. These radio communications are made more efficient by the use of "ten-codes," the numerical symbols that stand for particular conditions or instructions pertaining to company operations. Many of these codes are widely standardized, the most famous being the "ten-four" (10-04), which means "I understand you" or "I will comply," and figures prominently in police and firefighter shows on television and in citizens band radio traffic. Apart from that signal, the codes most frequently used in the company are:

10-08   In service
10-17   Ambulance call: lights and siren
10-16   Ambulance call: immediately, no lights or siren

10-19   Return to quarters
10-23   Arrived at scene
10-24   Assignment completed

Leaving the hospital after a run is usually the occasion for a preliminary debriefing. The crew members, who have not had an opportunity until now to talk together privately, compare notes on the run they have just made. In effect they construct a definition of the situation by going over the characteristics of the occurrence and sharing the different aspects they noted. They raise puzzling questions and seek answers from each other; they ask opinions about what they have surmised; each finds out if the other noticed a particular event or sight one of them found striking. If the run has been especially "good" they are in a sense rehearsing the story as they will tell it to the others when they get back to quarters. If the run was not worthy of comment, it will be evident in just that way—no one will comment on it. They will converse about other things or just ride silently. The run is by definition not good if it is not worth talking about. The EMTs do not always agree about a run. A new attendant may be eager to talk about the case of a patient with a foot lacerated by a power mower, while the crew chief, who has seen dozens of these accidents, will not find much of interest in the case unless the setting or the person is in some way unique.

10:32 AM
Tanner pulls into the alley behind the station and positions the ambulance to back into the parking area.
LOUIE *Want me to guide you in?*
TANNER *Don't bother. No problem.*
When the ambulance is stopped, Louie picks up the reports and climbs out. Just before Tanner switches off the rig's battery he makes a last call on the radio.
TANNER *Thirty-two is in quarters.*

3

in quarters

Crew Culture

Jase puts down the classified section in which he has been looking at ads for used canoes. He takes a swig of grape soda and shakes his head. "The worst I ever saw was on a run with the fire company in Jefferson. We got a call from the pumper to a private home. When we got there a graduation party was underway. We thought it must be the wrong address since everyone was having such a delightful time. Then we saw this fireman waving us in and motioning toward the downstairs. So there we are pushing our way through this crowded, laughing throng in the recreation room, not knowing what the hell's going on. Over in the far corner is another fireman waving frantically. We push our way through—"Excuse me, excuse me"—and we find a code! No shit! I was floored. These other people were paying absolutely no attention to what was going on. The guy's grandson was sitting calmly near the body eating his fucking dinner. I couldn't believe it! So we went to work down there in the corner with the music pounding away. I start bagging him and of course he vomits. So I clean out the mask by dumping the crap on one of the grandson's plates, just to relieve the fury. The grandson went on eating! It was like a Fellini movie. It scared the hell out of me to see these people completely unable to relate to reality." Jase pauses to answer another question before he starts reading again. Still shaking his head as though puzzled, he says, "No, we couldn't bring him around. It was too late."

In quarters, among the ambulance personnel, Jase's story was heard and understood somewhat differently than it would have been elsewhere. In quarters, crew culture prevails. Crew culture is not the same as the public culture of the wider society, or the occupational culture of the EMT, or even the organizational culture defined by the company's rules and policies. Crew culture is a little of each of these and a little more. It is a unique combination of values, concepts, assumptions, and customs that the personnel share with each other but not with outsiders. Crew culture consists of stories that are frequently retold, labels that categorize the world, favored explanations of human behavior, and expectations about how crew members are to behave. It is shaped and supported by the common interests of the crews, the conditions of their work, and the notable experiences they share. Each of these factors increases the social solidarity within the group, while at the same time diminishing the ties between group members and outsiders.

The Sources of Crew Culture

Common Interests

In at least one respect Station 2 crew culture is very close to the dominant public culture: it is oriented to young, white males. Only a few of the company's ambulance attendants have been female, fewer have been non-white, and rarely have any been older than thirty.[1] The quarters offer ample evidence of this orientation—"skin" magazines, weights and other exercise equipment, electronic gadgets, and now and then a cigar. Overflowing ashtrays, empty soda bottles, cups half filled with cold coffee, and crumpled cigarette packs contribute to an impression of the occupants' disdain for routine cleaning chores. Talk about cars, girls, sports, and drinking bouts ("choir practice") is common at Station 2. This homogeneity, the fact that they share these interests, draws the EMTs together. The mutual attraction is compounded by another common interest which separates them from their peers outside the company—their interest in caring for the sick and the injured.

For most people the basic work of medicine, direct contact with disease, disability, and trauma, is not very appealing. The fascination with death and injury that is evident in the crowds that surround every accident scene is a fascination that requires distance. The idea of handling a dead body, bandaging a deep wound, or immobilizing a compound fracture is unsettling and even repugnant to these crowds. The feelings of most people are probably expressed by the teenager who told an EMT, "I don't see how you can stand it. It seems so morbid."

The EMTs, too, are bothered by some parts of the work—the vomit, the soiled beds and clothing, the ugly sores, the decomposing bodies. These unpleasant parts they try to dismiss with the inattention that routine allows. Instead they focus on interesting experiences and the opportunities to contribute to a patient's well-being. In the midst of the messy reality of medical activity they find a satisfaction that is idealistic without being romantic. It is not easily described or often articulated. As an example, we can again listen to Jase, who tried to find words for it after he had helped the fire department paramedics work on a "code" who was successfully revived.

Here is the payoff for all this! When we got here that guy was gone. Just a bag of potatoes. And then they brought him back. He might be a walk-away. Just recover and walk out of the hospital. He came back fast. Usually they have to really sweat over a case, but he came back very fast. In with the "epi" and he was on his way back.[2] That was neat; just so neat! Didn't you think that was neat?

The public's uneasiness about sickness and death and the EMTs' inability to explain the attraction they find in working with such misery indicate the boundary of understanding that separates the crew culture from the public culture. The EMTs share their side of that boundary with other medical and health workers, but they are separated from most of the people even in that select category by the peculiar conditions of crew work and by the particular experiences that have become part of crew history.

Conditions of Work

The emergency work of ambulance companies (like that of fire companies) cannot be scheduled. Because the demand for service may come at any time, it is difficult to make shift changes efficiently. The duty crews may be finishing runs while the personnel from the next shift have already reported for work and are sitting in quarters on paid time waiting for the cars to return. An obvious way to increase the efficiency of the operation is to minimize the number of shift changes. As a result the EMTs more often than not work extended shifts, for example, twenty-four hours on duty and forty-eight hours off in sequence. It is true at least for private companies that ambulance personnel work more than forty hours per week and that their schedules rotate so that from week to week they work different days and/or different hours.

One of the consequences of these irregular schedules is the "jet lag" phenomenon. Our bodies operate according to a set of biological cycles or rhythms that are adjusted to each other, to our environment, and to our routine activities.[3] When our routines are upset in a significant way, as when we travel swiftly across several time zones, thus altering our relation to astronomical time, our biological rhythms become desynchronized and we experience a variety of unpleasant symptoms. Because ambulance crews are continually forced to alter their eating and sleeping times, their bodies are not able to maintain integrated patterns of biological rhythms.[4] It is reasonable to suspect that this physiological imbalance can have a direct effect on how the crews perform their duties. Sleep deprivation (either in quantity or in subjective quality), for example, has been associated with an increase in anxiety, irritability, suspicion, difficulty concentrating, inefficiency, and performance errors.[5] It would be interesting to know the relation of changes in work schedule or of the recent sleep history of ambulance personnel to vehicle accidents or to the quality of patient care.

The conditions of their work also subject ambulance attendants to *social dislocation,* the circumstance in which one's normal activities are out of phase with the dominant society's schedule for those activities. Night workers, for example, suffer social dislocation because, even though they might follow a regular, forty-hour work schedule each week, they must sleep during those hours when the rest of the world is transacting business—when the telephone is ringing, the children are coming home from school, the stores are open, and so forth.[6] Ambulance workers, because of their long shifts, must sleep at least part of the time during regular business hours. Because of this and because of their changing schedules, they are unable to participate in many events that are open to the majority of the public, a fact that contributes to the separation between crew culture and public culture.

Yet it is not only the unconventional timing of their work schedules that causes the social dislocation of the crews, it is also the unpredictability of their work obligations. Ambulance attendants are often called on short notice to fill someone else's shift. Last-minute vacancies on the duty roster occur in several circumstances; among the more important are personnel who leave with little or no notice,[7] sickness (including "mental health leaves" when the personnel simply feel incapable of facing the job), unanticipated family problems, exceptional recreational opportunities, transportation problems, and even oversleeping. Other events allow for advance planning of shift changes but still require that people alter their usual routines; examples of these are technical training programs, mandatory court appearances, vacations, and celebrations of weddings or birthdays.

Liberty Ambulance Company prefers that open shifts be covered by part-time employees. It costs the company less to reimburse part-timers, whose base salary is usually lower than that of regular employees, than to pay overtime to full-time workers. To promote their preferences, the owners keep a list of active part-time employees on the bulletin board at Station

2. The crews, however, typically find it more convenient to ask one of their regular colleagues to take an extra shift for them than to try to find a part-timer able and willing to work. The trading of shifts can create such a complicated set of schedules that it sometimes becomes the main topic of conversation in quarters.

There are at least three reasons why EMTs are willing to take on the extra disruption caused by sudden schedule changes. First, though not necessarily most important, the full-timers often are interested in the increased pay that comes with overtime. They are particularly interested if the extra shifts are convenient, that is, if they are immediately before or after one of their scheduled shifts, even though they may have to work thirty or more hours without a break. (Flash claimed the company record for longest tour of duty; he once worked 104 hours straight.) EMTs employed by private ambulance companies make little more than the minimum wage; they make ends meet by working long hours.

Second, there is an informal *code of reciprocity* within the company that prompts the personnel to fill in for one another.[8] In simple terms the code implies that since everyone is in need of help sometimes, everyone should be willing to be helpful whenever possible. Applied to this case, the code says that since anyone might eventually be in need of a substitute on short notice, one should be willing to fill in when it is reasonably convenient. The person who accepts an extra shift is in effect doing it as a favor to a co-worker and as a favor to the company; he thereby establishes both the indebtedness of a specific individual and a positive record with his employers. The helper's benefits are not limited to those who are specifically in debt to him, however; he also establishes general obligations within the social network of employees by earning the reputation of one who is "willing to help out."[9] The owners let their employees know that they are expected to be available to fill in from time to time when there is a special need; word gets around that a certain person who resists is considered a "hard ass." At the same time, one of the owners' favorite EMTs made it a principle not to take extra shifts but was not penalized.

The informal code provides a means for handling schedule crises through the exchange of favors. It is supported by a set of sanctions brought to bear on people who fail to reciprocate when a benefactor needs help. The offender is teased, criticized, and denounced by the other employees and can acquire a reputation that will exclude him from the support of his fellows. This reputation can also cause the employer to be more or less unpleasant if the employee accidentally damages one of the cars. At times the company itself can be considered unjust,[10] though the only recourse the offended party has is to cut back on subsequent investments of good will. Often it is difficult to establish exactly which party is failing to uphold its end of the implicit bargain.

Clark slammed down the blue phone. "Shit! Jack said he would come in and now he tells me he can't. Dandy said he would work if things really got tough, but he just finished an extra shift and you can't ask someone to come back after that. I am really pissed off! Everything was fine. I got you to replace me so I could leave early. Then at the last minute The Doctor had his wife call to say he had a test moved up so he has to study for it. He was probably afraid to call in himself. Then B.Z. didn't find anyone to replace The Doctor, even though that's his job as personnel supervisor. Now I have to stay over 'til we find someone to take The Doctor's place. And my wife and I have an appointment with the realtor to look at apartments in fifteen minutes. Shit! After I put in all kinds of overtime to help the company out, then they treat me like this. I am really pissed!

Third, and much less obvious, at least some of the EMTs have a commitment to their work, a sense of the urgency of the enterprise, that impels them to keep the cars running even when it is personally inconvenient. At Liberty, commitment seems to be greater for those who come from small towns and who have experience as volunteers. Because they feel both an obligation to their coworkers and pressure from their employers, it is easy to explain their behavior in terms of these forces and ignore the more subtle factor. Yet there are times when an individual will change his plans (which would have been an acceptable excuse for not returning),[11] even when he has no "debts" to repay, in order to fill an open shift. Prospective substitutes will give an affirmative response ("If you can't find anyone else, I'll come in, but I'd rather not."), even though a supervisor is calling rather than a coworker, and even if he could make up an excuse. In these instances the EMTs seem to be moved by a conviction that it is critical to keep the full roster of ambulances crewed and on the road.

The fact is that one car out of operation would probably not seriously affect the safety of the public,[12] and the crews are aware of this, as they show when they gripe about the lack of "good" runs. At the same time, there is the logical possibility that having enough cars operating could prevent a delay in response, which might make all the difference for a patient. Further, it would be strange if the crews did not feel there was an urgency about keeping the cars on the road. If they were to admit that their work was unimportant, few of them would be willing to accept the responsibilities of the job for so little compensation. Their belief in the importance of what they are doing gives them a reason for carrying out the work and puts them under pressure to make sure it is done properly. An ambulance without a crew is a symbol of the unimportance of the work, and there are almost always enough people who do not want to have that symbol displayed to keep the shifts filled.

This sense of urgency in ambulance work can also be inferred from the willingness of the personnel to put up with inconveniences in their everyday activities. A final comment from Jase, about his volunteer work, both describes some of the minor burdens EMTs accept as a matter of course and emphasizes the gap of understanding between crew culture and the public:

Families can't really understand the situation if they're not involved themselves. My parents are always wanting to know why I don't call more regularly. They can't appreciate how drained a person is after they get off work and how they have to wind down. They don't understand why I can't go right to sleep after a shift and then have lots of time to take care of my personal affairs. If I'm on call with the Jefferson Rescue Squad and we're having dinner at home and a call comes in, my mother will say, "Why don't you finish eating before you go?" It's just incomprehensible to me that she can't grasp that every second is important in an emergency. Or my father will criticize me for not letting my car warm up in the winter before taking off on a call. I know it ruins the car, but what are you going to do? This is why it's important to have the office staff go along on runs now and then. They get some idea of what the EMTs are going through. Then they can appreciate more why we have difficulty getting all the information sometimes.

The crew culture sets the EMTs apart not only from the public but from the office staff within the company and to some extent from the owners, even though they are EMTs themselves.

The impact of the company's social dislocation can be seen in the strain it causes in family life.[13] The effects are evident in several ways. First, although the owners, office personnel, and some part-time attendants are married, most of the full-time attendants who have been with the company for at least six months are single. Personnel who get married while with the company usually leave a few months later. Second, a few of the part-time EMTs have quit working with the company altogether because their families complained about the hours. They said they were particularly concerned about the children but that they could rarely get to see even their spouses, especially if they too were working. Third, it appears that some of the EMTs are able to use their work as an effective means of escaping from their families. They put in tremendous amounts of overtime, supposedly because they need the money, but they hang around quarters even when they are not working and sleep there at times when they are not on duty. At least one of these cases ended in divorce.

The social dislocation of ambulance workers not only interferes with their family life, it also limits the contacts they have with other people.

They are pressured to develop social ties with others who share their dislocation, some within the company and some outside it.[14] A surprising number of the EMTs hang around the quarters for a while after they have clocked out, talking, smoking, in some cases reading. A few arrive as much as an hour before they are due to clock in and join in the prevailing activity, even if it is nothing more than watching television.

Crew members see each other away from quarters; they attend concerts and sports events together, visit each other at home, hit the bars together, invite the whole roster of employees to bachelor parties and weddings. Out of this social activity friendships develop. The female employees eventually become romantically involved with the male crew members. However, many of these friendships seem to have shallow roots since people quickly lose contact when one of them leaves the company. This characteristic suggests that the relationships are limited to the convenience of employment and thus may be a consequence of social dislocation.

The relationships the crews establish with hospital workers are probably due as much to limited contacts as to common interests, since some of the couples formed by the relationships eventually leave medical work altogether. Further, hospital workers, along with fast-food servers and gas station attendants, are about the only people crews see regularly on the night shifts or when they are busy. It is important to note that most of the ED admitting staffs and nurses are female, while nearly all the EMTs are male. That the hospital personnel reciprocate the EMTs' interest in establishing personal contacts is indicated to some extent by their inviting the EMTs to join in occasional informal social events.[15] The relationships that develop from such contacts sometimes become romantic and in a few cases have resulted in marriage.

Common Experiences

Crew culture develops out of shared experiences generated by the character as well as the conditions of ambulance work. Two kinds of work-related experiences are important: the ordinary and recurring experiences that shape the worker's general view of ambulance services and of society, and the specific experiences that are remembered as extraordinary events.

Ambulance personnel, like other public service workers, share not only the routine concerns of their jobs but also the opportunity to get an uncommon view of society. They see more of the backstage of social life than is permitted to others. They regularly come upon people who are in distress and panic, who are unable to sustain the normal "front" of competence and civility.[16] Very often what they see is an unflattering picture of humanity; what they are likely to remember are the least complimentary details of that picture.[17] They recognize the signs of child abuse, witness the brutality of alcoholics toward those who care about them, move through the filthy conditions of poverty, endure the whining complaints of the privileged, hear the shifting excuses of drunken drivers, notice how the hospitals ignore or deal abruptly with certain patients, watch the police cursing the people they apprehend.

It is difficult for the crews to describe in words the flavor of these events without having them seem flat, fragmentary, and trivial. The public carries a polite image of society that can only rarely make room for the discordant themes the crews want to express. At the same time, because they are so much aware of the disjunction between these two views of society, the ambulance workers need to talk about it. They therefore turn to those who can understand and appreciate what they feel. They chat with police and firefighters from time to time, but the most accessible and sympathetic ears belong to their colleagues within the company.

An important part of the conversations about work among the crews is a folklore consisting of stories about specific experiences of company personnel. These stories are polished and exaggerated as they are retold, and details are added from different occasions as though they were part of the same event. The stories are valued for the shocking elements they contain; the more horrendous, the better. Their content ranges from the mundane (the expected firing of an employee) to the dramatic (a shoot-out in an alley). There are stories about the messiest corpse, the most tragic automobile accident, the scariest psycho, the grossest violation of ethics by a competing company, the most embarrassing situation, the stupidest move by the rescue squad, the most unfeeling family, and so on.

There are several reasons for storytelling among the EMTs. One of the most obvious is their frequent need for *debriefing.*[18] The need depends on the nature of the run they have just completed. If the run was routine, they come into quarters quietly and deflect the attention of the people there by reporting, for example, that they just "hauled a wino to detox" (the detoxification unit at County Hospital). If, on the other hand, the run was interesting in some way, the crew will begin talking about it as soon as they come through the door—"Jesus! You shoulda seen that place! Garbage up to your knees and no lights! This woman was down in a back corner and out of her skull. . . ." The other EMTs are likely to respond with questions or stories about similar experiences. Talking provides a way for the crew to work off the tension built up on the run, and the response of the others eases the emotional impact by fitting the experience into a broader context. In the telling, the crews work out their fear and anger and, perhaps too rarely, celebrate their triumphs. Especially troubling events will sometimes trigger more intense discussions, tinged with philosophy or theology, about how people can tolerate filthy conditions or how a man can beat up his small daughter.

Some of these stories are *informational* in that they convey useful knowledge about specific conditions or general procedures. A story of one car's forced detour enlightens the rest of the crews about a closed street; a story about a CHF (congestive heart failure) patient who would not tolerate the oxygen mask suggests a way to deal with the problem; a story of a gurgling patient who could not be suctioned because the checkout crew had not set up the suctioning unit reminds everyone to be thorough in their routines.

Another reason for the stories is that they are considered *entertainment*. Time often hangs heavy in quarters and the sharing of stories becomes a pleasant way to spend otherwise tedious periods of waiting. Some of the stories clearly have no other value than the possibility of raising a laugh. One such story was about Car 30, which was smashed up as soon as it was put into service. After a month in the body shop and an extra careful inspection of its mechanical systems, the rig was brought back to the station to be equipped and have new stick-on identification applied. When a quart of oil was added it ran out onto the floor—the filler tube hadn't been reattached! When the rig was driven out to go on duty, it stalled only a few blocks from the station, the flashers and turn signals failed, and smoke began pouring out of the steering column! The driver radioed for a wrecker. "Harold [the owner] must have jumped out of his skin. A mile on the road and it has to be towed."

In addition to these benefits of storytelling, there are some consequences that are less well recognized but equally important. The stories contribute to the *socialization* of the newer EMTs; that is, they provide an orientation to emergency medical work that is not available in books and courses. They give some idea of what to expect with one's first DOE ("dead on entry," which refers to a corpse) or one's first visit to the "cop shop" (district jail). They alert the EMTs to certain addresses ("Last night we got a 3:00 AM call to 1515 Longview. Fucking three in the morning. You've been up there to the 'crazy house' haven't you, Gundy?") or to certain people ("We hauled Noah Blue again yesterday. Same old problem—can't breathe. He's taken up chewing tobacco. His beard has a brown stripe down the middle now. I made him hold the big pan in his lap all the way. He looked like he was going to throw up; I think he swallowed some of that shit. St. Chris's doesn't want him back there any more. They can't do anything for him.").

Finally, the stories create *solidarity* among the crews. They are all told from the point of view of the EMT and for the most part derive their humor from the antics of outsiders. Knowing the stories and being able to add appropriate embellishments is a sign of belonging.[19] Having stories told about one's own adventures is a further validation of one's status within the crew culture.

It is less evident what contribution is made by the theories that are passed around as common knowledge and become part of the folklore. One hears many generalizations: accidents are more numerous on Saturdays; warm days are especially busy; the number of "crazy calls" (odd or unusual patients) goes up when there is a full moon. It is not clear whether any of these theories are true, but some are certainly false. The prediction that after St. Patrick's Day crews would be hauling lots of "the miseries" (hangovers) was proved wrong. The theory that no one in the company wanted to work out of the new quarters on the edge of the ghetto was wrong; in spite of the public theory, nearly everyone had a private reason for wanting to work out of that station. Theories and opinions sometimes develop into extended discussions that wax and wane over several days without resolution:

Four vehicles pull up to an intersection with a four-way stop at the same time—a fire engine, a police car, an ambulance, and a post office truck. Which one has the right of way? Correct, the post office truck!
Bullshit!
No, that's the law. . . .

These theories and the discussions that examine them seem to serve as touchstones against which the crews can test their own experience and knowledge, gathering evidence and arguments in support or in opposition. They express issues that give some shape to the conversations in quarters.

Thus, there exists a crew culture that separates company personnel from those who don't belong. It not only distinguishes them from outsiders, it also helps to maintain the morale and efficiency of the crews. The content of this crew culture is evident in the issues discussed throughout the rest of this book.

The Texture of Time

Life in quarters is governed by outside forces. Events over which the crews have no control determine how they will spend the work shift. These events upset their most carefully conceived plans and intrude on their most private acts. But unlike the assembly line worker, who is held to a mechanically steady pace, the ambulance worker is subject to fluctuations in the intensity of work. Sometimes the EMT longs for a moment to rest; just as often he longs for something, anything, to happen.

External Control

The EMTs on duty are on an electronic leash. In quarters they can be reached by telephone; when they leave they carry a pager that can signal them to make radio contact with their dispatcher. Any activity—eating a meal, going to the toilet, having the ambulance refueled—can be interrupted. Since the rationale for organizing an ambulance service is to insure a prompt response, there are no acceptable excuses for delaying the reaction to an emergency call.

The EMTs most often talk about interruptions in connection with sleep. There are predictable expressions of amazement whenever someone reports having rested undisturbed through the first shift (midnight to 8:00 AM). The folklore even includes stories about the disorientation of a crew that returned from a run at 2:00 AM and slept until noon the next day. The stories are of interest because the crews consider them exceptional. They pessimistically assume that a night crew will not be able to sleep more than two hours at a stretch.

The crews use a variety of strategies to protect themselves against the most inconvenient intrusions.[20] For example, they often observe the informal rule of "last car in, last car out." If Squad 32 returns to quarters after completing a run and finds two other duty crews already there, Squad 32 assumes the others will take the next two runs.[21] The crew members have, in effect, some *protected time* in which to eat, clean up, or whatever, However, two emergency calls in quick succession can eliminate their advantage in a few minutes and put them back in the realm of the unpredictable.

At other times the crews will cover for each other without regard for the number or recency of runs each has made. Two crews will handle all the calls while the third, for example, has a meal. This arrangement may be agreed to among the duty crews themselves; more often it includes the co-operation of the dispatcher, who recognizes the third unit as being temporarily "out of service." Even the support of all the working personnel, however, cannot provide a complete safeguard. If there is a rash of calls, the protected crew will be called into action.[22] In one instance the members of a crew went out of service to order a fast-food meal at a fish-and-chips shop. After they had paid but before their order had arrived, they got a call. The counterman said he would hold their order. An hour later they picked up the food but got another run before they could eat. An hour later they returned to quarters with the food but were called out immediately. An hour later they reheated the food in a microwave oven but were called out before they could eat it. An hour later, before they left quarters on another run, they threw the food away.

Apparently as a result of their having learned that even protected time is tentative at best, the most experienced EMTs have taken a somewhat fatalistic attitude toward scheduling meals. The crew chiefs advise the newer personnel to grab a bite when they feel like eating, since there is no way to predict when a call will interrupt them.

In extreme cases units may resort to *stretching the run* in order to find a free minute. This means they simply postpone informing the dispatcher that they are clear of their last obligation. The dispatcher assumes they are busy at the hospital and assigns calls to other units. But if the pressure is great enough, the dispatcher will use the pager to initiate contact with a crew that has not yet "cleared." While one crew member finishes the report to the emergency department, the other calls base and receives instructions for the next run. At times the tech may be forced to make up the cot in the back of the ambulance while they are running hot to the next emergency.

Work Rhythms

Ambulance work is, like military service, an alternation between hurrying and waiting. The EMTs on duty are never free of the threat of a sudden alarm. They are always on "hold." They can never fully relax. They are startled from their shallow naps by the ringing of the phone. Yet for long periods they are forced to do little more than wait. They cannot be far from the red telephone or from the ambulance. They find it impossible to occupy themselves with anything that cannot be dropped at a moment's notice, and difficult to do anything that requires concentration.[23] In an instant the requirements of their situation can alter from a need for passive tolerance to a need for swift and purposeful action.

There is no such thing as a normal work shift, according to the crews. Tours of duty are described by extremes. They are either "busy" or "slow." These terms are useful descriptions not only of shifts, but also of the kinds of time that make up the work life of the ambulance attendant. Duty time is busy when the EMT is actively engaged in emergency medical service, in making runs. Time is slow when the EMT is waiting to make a run. In the company a crew averages a patient transport about once every two hours. There are "no transport" calls and "head to" calls in addition, and runs are more numerous during the daylight and twilight hours, but each kind of time represents roughly half the working day. (See Appendix B.)

Except in unusual circumstances, a run is always *busy time*. The emphasis is on action rather than reflection. Busy time is dense in that there are many foci of attention and many responsibilities to be dealt with at once.

There seem to be too few minutes in which to do everything that is necessary. When the busy time is over, one is amazed that it is so late. On a run,
for example, the combination of many duties—running hot and locating
the address, dealing with many witnesses and reporters and assessing the
patient, monitoring vital signs and doing the paperwork—creates the
potential for system overload. There is too much information to be pro-
cessed by one person; the EMT must resort to techniques for controlling
the rate of inputs.

The EMTs cope with busy time partly by anticipating it. Being familiar
with the location of equipment in the ambulance and trauma box, arrang-
ing the forms in a special way in the tripbook, knowing what forms can be
filled out beforehand and what afterward, developing efficient ways of
combining questions with the checking of vital signs, all help the EMT to
get through especially demanding times. The EMT also develops selective
attention—ignoring everything but cross traffic and street signs when running hot and concentrating on one or two witnesses when gathering information. Occasionally the driver will take it slowly if the patient is not critical, or even stop around the corner to allow for a blood pressure check, if
the tech needs time to complete his assessment or fill out the reports for the
hospital.

Slow time is the time of the prisoner. Confined to a too familiar space,
one scans for items of interest or naps without being tired. Thought processes are on idle. The passage of time itself becomes an obsession expressed in repeated glances at the clock. On a normal day slow time in
quarters is broken up by the arrival and departure of other crews as well as
by one's own runs; on a slow shift there are too few of these occurrences to
provide adequate markers of the progress of the day. While slow time is
usually a matter of waiting in quarters for a run, it also includes sitting in the
ambulance on a strategic street corner while covering for another company, making a long distance transfer of an uninteresting patient, or even
carrying drunks to the detoxification center.

The EMTs cope with slow time in a variety of ways. Naturally enough,
conversations fill much of the time, although they eventually become predictable. It is only partially in jest that rookies are greeted as "new blood,"
for they do provide new viewpoints and new subjects for conversation.
Some of the personnel work on company business, loading the Coke
machine, washing the rigs, doing the laundry (towels and blankets), and
cleaning the quarters. Most of these activities are taken up only with the
encouragement of the supervisors. Other people write letters or make personal telephone calls to the extent that the public setting will allow. The
predominant standbys, however, are reading and watching television. In
the space of a few months the reading matter displayed in quarters varies
considerably, ranging from *Hustler* and *People* magazines through books

on the philosophies and techniques of the martial arts to *The Rise and Fall of the Third Reich.* On the medical side, specialized publications, such as *The EMT Journal* and *Emergency,* are read regularly. Popular books on medicine (for example, *Bellevue*) turn up, and occasionally someone can be seen studying the side effects of drugs in the *Physicians' Desk Reference.* The television set is on nearly all the time. Comedies and serials are favored, perhaps because they can be enjoyed even if one's viewing is interrupted. "M.A.S.H.," the series about a military hospital unit, is one of the favorites of the crews and is affectionately referred to as a "training film." Finally, when all else fails, eating becomes a way to pass the time. Going out to eat is a valid excuse for getting some exercise, but even the soft drink machine and the honor-system candy supply in quarters get a good workout in especially slow periods.

Making the transition from one kind of time to the other is a serious problem for the crews. The lethargy of slow time seems to infect and retard them when they are called out. They move promptly but forget things, confuse the address, have trouble locating their jackets. Their lack of sharpness could ultimately affect the quality of patient care they render. The transition in the other direction, from busy time to slow time, may be equally difficult for the EMT but it does not directly affect the patient. If a run has been at all interesting, the EMTs are likely to be "high" and ready to talk about it. They move about restlessly and complain when there is no action. It takes a while to adjust to doing nothing. The transition in either direction is probably more difficult when the personnel are tired. One of the skills new EMTs must learn is to adjust to the rhythm of activity and thereby control their feelings of frustration.

Individuals seem to differ as to whether they prefer busy time or slow time. Flash often asks the dispatcher to give his car as many runs as possible, and he is quick to volunteer to cover for other squads when they want to go out of service. Other people claim they wouldn't care if they didn't have to go out at all during the shift. However, there may be limits to human tolerance for a particular kind of time. After twelve hours of having no calls, for example, even the indifferent begin to look around for something to happen. In quarters at such a time nearly everyone becomes snappish and argumentative. Similar conduct is evident when the squads have been busy for a sustained period. EMTs shout at ED personnel, complain about the dispatcher, and toss their uncompleted paperwork (hindered by the frantic pace) into a jumbled heap on the cab floor. In this case the squad members become allies against the outsiders and their unrealistic demands. Where the problem is too little work, there is no compensatory strengthening of social solidarity. The nature of ambulance work is such that the personnel have very little opportunity to regulate its tempo and thus to moderate the consequences of excess.

The Five Finger Discount

One of the most striking examples of crew culture is an activity the EMTs refer to as "the five finger discount"—the unauthorized acquisition of hospital supplies. It is a pattern of behavior not found in the public culture. Indeed, the crews, including those who are not actively involved, cooperate in keeping it secret from outsiders. It is not necessarily unique to the company, although it can exist only under certain conditions.[24] Quite possibly it is as much a consequence of the motivations and organization of ambulance workers in general as of the peculiarities of the situation of company personnel.

In some instances the five finger discount is morally ambiguous; in other cases it is obviously illegal. For example, when a hospital transfers a patient and provides the crew with a sterile forceps to be used should anything happen to the patient's chest tube, it is not clear what should be done with the instrument at the end of the run. Doubtless it will end up in the instrument holster of one of the EMTs. The crews do nothing to resolve this ambiguity since it is profitable for them. On the other hand, when an attendant picks up a bottle of irrigation water from the hospital storeroom and slips it under the rumpled blanket on the cot he is wheeling, his stealth betrays his understanding that the act is in some sense improper. He seems to realize most people would consider it theft.

Company personnel are aware of the unauthorized lifting of equipment and supplies; the topic comes up occasionally in conversations in quarters. However, only about one-fourth of the workers are directly involved in either securing or accepting discounted items. Experienced EMTs are the active participants. Nearly all the discounters are crew chiefs, with only two techs (both of whom have since become crew chiefs) taking part. The discounters are all people for whom emergency medical services are an important focus of their attention both on the job and off.

This focus is prominent in the purpose the EMTs give for lifting supplies—to improve the quality of emergency medical care. The supplies are neither sold for money nor used for pleasure. Some items, such as the forceps mentioned above, become part of an EMT's personal gear. Other items are used to supplement the equipment provided by the company, as can be seen in this description:

During checkout of the rigs at the beginning of the second shift [8:00 AM to 4:00 PM] we heard Barb tell Jardine she needed some Tempo-dots, a throwaway temperature indicator not issued by the company but carried by some of the EMTs. On the way back to Station 2 after the shift, Louie asked Jardine if he were going to make delivery. Jar-

dine pulled a box of Tempodots from his squad jacket and handed them to Louie with the comment, "I like to keep my customers happy." He also pulled out a still-packaged cervical collar, though we had not used one during that shift. Louie looked it over and said he would take it for his own first aid kit.

Probably most five finger acquisitions are used in private "trauma boxes"—elaborate first aid kits the EMTs carry in their cars to deal with emergencies they might encounter off duty. Some of these kits include splints and backboards, and they are nearly as well equipped in smaller items as the ambulances.

I was looking for a pediatric [small size] cervical collar to show to my son's kindergarten class. Lyle said the company didn't have any but that he would lend me one from his car. "It was just lying around St. Christopher's for about five weeks so I decided it was meant for me." Lyle has two kits in the back of his car. He says one is for general first aid and the other is for major trauma.

The personnel seem sometimes to suspect that these preparations are excessive. Once, while the crews were talking about the theft a few months earlier of the company's new and expensive heart monitor, they began humorously speculating about the possibility of an EMT riding around with a $5,000 "Life Pac" in his car on the chance that he'll come across a stray cardiac emergency.

   Among the beneficiaries of the five finger discount are the volunteer service groups with which many of the EMTs are associated. The volunteers furnish some of their own equipment (forceps, scissors, penlights, and so forth), which in the case of company EMTs might have been five-fingered. Beyond that, the groups usually accept donations of materials, and the crews are inclined to help out in this regard whenever they can, as the following suggests:

We were delivering an ETOH [drunk] to detox when Jardine got hung up just inside the downstairs door. There were stacks of cartons of large sterile dressings in the hallway. Jardine could hardly restrain himself from tossing one into the back of the ambulance. He said Tanner could use some of those when his volunteer rescue squad unit covered their county fair. But it would look bad if we had that thing in the rig and got a call before we could unload it at Station 2.

My notes from a few days later include this:

*On the way back from Zion [Hospital] after our first run, I noticed a
bag of Ringer's [solution for intravenous therapy] on the floor of the
cab along with some other equipment. Jardine must have gotten it at
the hospital. That's why he was so eager to take the cot downstairs
while I was finishing the reports on the patient. He said he would turn
the stuff over to Tanner for his group to use at the fair. From Jardine's
point of view, the hospital received a bag of Ringer's with the patient
and therefore should be prepared to furnish us with a replacement. His
argument is all right as far as it goes, but we didn't furnish the Ringer's
in the first place, the nursing home did. This way the patient will probably be charged twice, once by the nursing home and once by the hospital, while an Explorer Scout first aid kit at some county fair will have
a "free" IV setup.*

It is important to recognize that the crews do not practice the five finger
discount on company supplies. Whether it is because of the risk of losing
their jobs or because it seems too easy, there is no raiding of the stores at
Station 2. There is plenty of opportunity, since each EMT has a key to
quarters and most of the supplies are readily available for restocking the
ambulances. In fact, far from stealing from the company, personnel sometimes pick up extra nasal cannulas or oxygen masks or cervical collars and
add them to the regular inventory. There is no evidence at all that the company knows about these contributions or rewards them. Certainly there is
no public encouragement of the practice.

The five finger operators have developed an elaborate set of justifica-
tions for their behavior. Jardine in particular maintains that the good intentions of the actor mitigate any apparent violations of ethics or law. The
main points of the justification are that:

1. Since the city and county are underwriting a considerable part of the
   emergency medical system and a large additional amount is written
   off for charity, the hospital supplies for the most part belong to the
   taxpayers.
2. Providing extra equipment for the EMTs improves their morale and
   makes their work more effective, thus improving medical care.
3. Enabling EMTs to be equipped to handle off-duty emergencies extends the coverage of emergency services and thus improves medical
   care.
4. The improvement of emergency medical care lowers the overall cost
   of injuries and thus saves everyone money in the long run.

Jardine put it more succinctly in one of his discourses: "People wouldn't
complain if one of Tanner's group saved their lives, would they?"

There is more than a hint of Robin Hood in this activity—a noble cause, a service to the common man, a risky enterprise. The EMTs are involved in a grass-roots transfer of payments in which they take over the allocation of goods while someone else bears the cost. Five-fingered supplies are supposedly liberated so they will be more accessible to the wider community; they are paid for by a mixture of taxes, insurance premiums, and out-of-pocket patient expenditures. Like the escapades of Robin Hood, the five finger discount offers a challenge and an opportunity for excitement. The operators eagerly display their successes and recount close shaves and the audacious fabrications they offer to hospital personnel. Jardine, who is probably the chief practitioner of the art, has said he gets a kick out of it and even goes so far as to admit a fascination with the idea of being a "wheelman" or a "hit man" for "the mob." In a curious contradiction he also expresses great indignation at the practice of policemen accepting "freebies" (free meals, tickets, and other items of value) from those who might expect favors in return. "It can't help but compromise their position. I wouldn't do it."

The five finger discount is possible because of the vagueness of the system of which the company is a part. It is understood, by some at least,[25] that the hospitals will charge emergency patients for supplies used during the prehospital phase (rescue squads and ambulances) of their care, and the ambulances will charge only a flat fee for transportation and skilled care anywhere within the county. The rescue squads and ambulances are allowed to replace their expendable supplies from hospital stores. However, there is slippage in this system. For example, a rescue squad, as first responders, might use a disposable oxygen line and mask to stabilize a patient. When they turn the patient over to the private ambulance for transport to a hospital, they may forget to ask for a replacement. The ambulance crew might then ask the hospital for a replacement, implying that they originally furnished the mask used on the patient. They thus acquire a "free" piece of equipment which can be added either to the company supplies or to their own private kits. Meanwhile, the rescue squad will discover they are short a mask and replace it from County Hospital's stores. The taxpayers and the patient each pay for a mask, though only one was used.

The five finger discount can be interpreted in more than one way. We can understand it as an attempt by workers to introduce some excitement into what have become routine and boring activities. Or we can understand it as an opportunity for people who are relatively powerless to get some satisfaction from working the system. But along with these interpretations we ought to realize that the discounters are engaging in deviant ways of *furthering their occupational mission*. The products of their deviance are channelled into emergency medical work, along with equipment purchased with their own funds and along with the time they volunteer.

The discounters signal the importance of their work by taking risks for it; they justify the risks by asserting the importance of their work. This dedication that stretches a job into a mission is more characteristic of a profession than of the kinds of blue-collar work associated with low pay and little public recognition. Perhaps the five finger discount shows, among other things, that ambulance workers are blue-collar professionals.

blue-collar professionals

Recruitment and Training

EMERGENCY MEDICAL TECHNICIAN: Wisconsin state or nationally registered. Part time or full time with benefits. Call 376-2601 Mon.-Fri. 8-4. equal opportunity employer

ATTENDANT: ambulance, full-time and part-time positions, insurance, benefits, only EMTs need apply. 453-2092.

These advertisements are a sign of the changing times in ambulance work. In the mid-1960s the private ambulance companies could probably pick up all the attendants they wanted by word of mouth. If they were forced to advertise, the only qualifications they were likely to cite were minimum age, driving record, and perhaps a chauffeur's license. First aid skills were clearly secondary and could be picked up either through experience or by such training as the company might offer for the sake of appearances or to satisfy minimal regulations.[1]

The ads appeared in metropolitan papers in 1978 and 1980. By specifying that it is EMTs they want, these companies are giving primary attention to the workers' qualifications in basic life support. EMT status is granted by the individual states as a result of a candidate's performance on either the state's own tests or on the standardized National Registry examinations. Some states require National Registry accreditation of candidates before they can be licensed.[2] This means that "ambulance attendant" now is a formally recognized occupational position that cannot be filled by anyone off the street. That change explains why the advertisements refer to "insurance" and "benefits." The supply of qualified personnel is much smaller than formerly, and employers must now compete to fill their rosters.

In addition to receiving formal recognition for his occupation through government regulations, the ambulance attendant has been given a public image in the popular media. The most dramatic of the media depictions are television shows, particularly "Emergency" (which appeared in reruns as "Emergency One") and "240-Robert." News and TV specials—through their coverage of CPR, paramedic programs, and trauma centers—have also contributed to increased public awareness of EMTs. More directly to the point, newspaper supplements on employment opportunities now list emergency medical technicians as a work category.[3]

Further, both commercial and "professional" interests attest to the distinctive role of the ambulance attendant. Along with the development and merchandising of new medical equipment for emergency services, an entire line of products is aimed at the self-conscious EMT. Coffee mugs, necklaces, T-shirts ("EMTs Do It on the Move!"), rings, license plate frames, cigarette lighters, jogging shorts, tie tacs, belt buckles, and solar-compass watches, all emblazoned with the star-of-life symbol and labeled "emergency medical technician," are offered to the occupants of this new position. New periodicals aimed at the EMT carry both commercial advertisements and news and feature articles on the state of the art. A survey in early 1980 found a surprisingly large number of publications directed toward EMS, which was then scarcely more than ten years old. It counted thirty-three journals and magazines, twenty-seven national newsletters, and forty-six regional newsletters related to EMS.[4] The professional interests of the EMT have been taken up by associations organized at the state and national levels for the most part, though a few local and regional groups are active too. With little effort, a working EMT today can be carrying a state license, a National Registry number, a National Association of Emergency Medical Technicians (NAEMT) membership card, and a state EMT association card.

As if to add a final seal of approval to the enterprise, the American Medical Association in 1979 approved emergency medicine as its twenty-third official specialty. A year later an emergency medicine physician was selected as a candidate for the National Aeronautics and Space Administration's space shuttle program.[5]

Yet in spite of this accumulating recognition of his distinctive role, the EMT (or ambulance attendant) has not achieved an unambiguous place within our social institutions. Not only does the public confuse the titles of ambulance workers by using "paramedic" too broadly, even within the occupation there is a lack of consistency in the terminology employed. The use of the star-of-life symbol, which is by now widely associated with EMS, is only laxly regulated.[6] Moreover, the lack of attention given to emergency medicine by related fields, such as medical sociology, shows that EMS is not yet seen as having an importance equal to that of the more traditional areas of medicine.[7] The upshot is confusion about the status of the EMT, confusion for the EMT himself and for the society he seeks to serve.

While in recent years there has been significant upgrading of ambulance work and ambulance workers, the changes are not yet complete. The EMT is now expected to bear a great deal of responsibility and to perform with competence and even dedication. At the same time his position in both the health care system and the occupational structure of sociey is marginal. To the workers, the rewards do not seem to be commensurate with the requirements of the job, and this inconsistency eventually has an effect on their behavior.

The Blue-Collar Professional

There are both insiders' and outsiders' views of a job. Outsiders, with their fragmentary knowledge, evaluate jobs by comparing them according to general properties, such as pay, hours, attractiveness of the work place, and head or hand work. Insiders, though they are very much aware of these comparisons, are also influenced by the character of the work, because of their concrete experiences. These two ways of viewing a job—the status of the occupation and the character of the work—do not necessarily agree. Many jobs that appear to the outsider to be highly desirable are, to the insider, barely tolerable, and vice versa. Ambulance work seems to be a case where the two views do not agree, where the insider's estimate is higher than that of the outsider.

The Status of the Occupation

We can think of status as a combination of prestige, power, and pay. Being ranked very high in terms of any one of these three criteria usually means overall high status. It is probably safe to say that ambulance work is not ranked high on any of them. Moreover, the workers are aware of the status of their occupation, and this awareness affects their morale on the job and their decisions about when to leave it.

The EMTs see scant evidence that they are held in high regard by society. Most people give little thought to ambulance services generally, and almost no one recognizes the formal position of the EMT specifically. If the public gives a passing thought to the work, it is likely to concern its morbid nature or its cost. This sense of the low prestige of ambulance work is evident in the attitude of a university student (known as "The Doctor"), who worked part time with Liberty Ambulance Company:

The Doctor hated to drive by the university, which is in our service area. He would crouch down in the seat and lean his head back out of sight of the window. "Jesus, I hope we don't get a call to campus. I don't want anyone to see me. I don't tell anyone I drive an ambulance. I don't know why exactly, but people wouldn't understand. They think this is just a nothing job. I even feel awkward going into a fast-food joint wearing this Liberty Ambulance patch. It's like being a walking billboard."

Employees of private ambulance companies hear a lot of griping about the cost of their services. In addition, Liberty employees are aware of a petition drive to drop the privates from the city EMS system and to return the responsibility for ambulance services to the untrained but "free" personnel of the Metropolitan Police Department. They even discovered that signatures were being gathered at the service station where the company bought 500 gallons of gas each week.[8] These activities of the public sector signal a clear dissatisfaction with, if not an utter disregard for, the position of the EMT.

The prestige of the occupation is affected, too, by the fact that more than half of the active EMTs are volunteers.[9] The high proportion of volunteers calls into question the social value of the activity and the level of accomplishment of full-time practitioners. How important can a job be if we rely for the most part on charity to handle it? How much pride can a paid EMT have in his occupation if most of his peers do the same thing for nothing? The crews are aware of this strain because most of them serve as volunteers too. They admit the irony of getting paid for the same work they otherwise volunteer for, but they say, "I'll take the money. I'm not proud."

The status of an occupation is ranked not only by its contribution to society or its formal requirements, but also by the kinds of people who are attracted to it. That is, it is not just that the work ennobles the worker; the prestige of the worker can ennoble the work. For example, "male" occupations are accorded higher status than "female" occupations. In the United States the occupation of physician has high prestige and about 90 percent of the practitioners are male;[10] in Russia nearly 80 percent of physicians are female and the medical profession has a markedly lower status.[11] Occupations selected by largely middle- and upper-class populations are likely to be accorded more prestige than other occupations, regardless of their social value or the skills they require.

The apparently low status of ambulance work is to some extent a consequence of the low status of the people who have been associated with it. For a long while ambulance attendants were losers who had missed out on their first choices and had fallen into a job that required little of them except the ability to lift a cot or to drive a station wagon.[12] Though the public may still hold this traditional impression, the more recent recruits to ambulance work are from a different stratum of society. The role of EMT now demands a greater measure of intelligence, self-control, and flexibility than was formerly the case. To qualify as an EMT requires a person to invest considerable time in classwork, to understand medical terminology and medical models, and to pass both written and practical examinations. The examinations are no longer simply for show. By 1980 nearly 15 percent of those who had taken the National Registry examinations had failed them, and in some cases as many as 50 percent of the EMT candidates drop out of the classes before they get to the exams.[13]

The Liberty employees are a diverse lot. While most of them favor rock, Tanner occasionally cruises around in the ambulance listening to classical music on the radio. Many of the books read in quarters are popular novels, but Flash often reads thick books of nonfiction. One employee may pass around his collection of homemade pornography, while another spends his days off practicing rock climbing. But these people are certainly not the dregs of society. Only about one in six of the Liberty personnel have held no full-time jobs before starting with the company, and these are college students or people just out of high school. The rest held steady jobs, usually higher paying, before they decided to work "on the cars." Some of them joined because they preferred the hours; others were looking for a change; still others were caught by layoffs and simply moved from part-time to full-time work with the company. The great majority of the employees had some education beyond the high school level.[14] When they left the company, the workers moved to such jobs as construction supervisor, auto parts department manager, industrial equipment sales representative, commercial pilot, physician's aide, emergency department technician, travel agent, computer programmer, paramedic, commercial art designer, furniture finisher, registered nurse, and firefighter.

This improvement in the attributes of ambulance attendants might eventually help increase the status of the occupation. For the moment, however, there is sufficient lag in the public's understanding of what is involved in ambulance work that the occupation continues to receive little prestige.

What the ambulance worker lacks in prestige he certainly does *not* make up for in power. The other workers with whom he must cooperate in the course of his duties usually outrank him in formal authority. Medical personnel in emergency departments, for example, are inclined to belittle the contribution of ambulance attendants. The EMTs, both the privates and the fire department rescue squads, complain that the ED staffs pay too little attention to their reports on patients. Because the EMTs are trained to appreciate the importance of the prehospital phase of care, they see the relative disinterest of the medical personnel as a downgrading of ambulance work. Part of the neglect by the hospital workers may be a continuation of the old conception that an ambulance is nothing more than a fast conveyance. Part may be rooted in a particular conception of what produces good patient care, a conception summarized by the medical student who said of EMTs, "With so little training, I don't see how they could offer more than a Bible and a Bandaid."

Liberty and the other private companies in Metropolis have a special problem, because the fire department is the first responder and is in control of the EMS system. At one of the company in-service training programs, the commissioner of health lectured the EMTs on the facts of life:

The law in this county is very clear. The authority for emergency medical services is with the fire chief. On the scene of an emergency in this city, the private EMT is officially under the authority of even the lowest, untrained firefighter. And I don't see any prospect of that law being changed.

As though being relegated to this powerless status were not enough, the privates are aware that even the EMTs within the fire department lack significant authority and position. For example, if they want to move up through the ranks, they, including the paramedics (EMT-Ps), must leave their specialty and advance strictly as firefighters. Because of this promotion system, and because rescue squad duty is seen as unheroic and exhausting,[15] the department people shy away from it, and even the EMTs

Table 4-1
COMPARISON OF PAY RATES
FOR SELECTED OCCUPATIONS, 1979

Occupation	Reported Hourly Wage
Medical technologist (laboratory)	$8.75
Supermarket cashier	7.00 +
Registered nurse (starting)	6.00–6.50
Furnace maintenance worker	5.50
Security guard	5.36
Licensed practical nurse	4.25 +
School crossing guard	4.21
EMERGENCY MEDICAL TECHNICIAN (private company)	3.85
Minimum wage	3.10

among them prefer to think of themselves as firefighters. There are very few occasions when the authority of an EMT extends to anyone other than the patient.

Perhaps the clearest and most influential indicator of an occupation's status is the rate of pay. According to this measure, the EMT ranks fairly low. Yet members of the middle classes express surprise when they learn how little EMTs are paid. Popular conceptions have the ambulance driver in the same stratum as other service workers, such as policemen and garbage collectors.[16] Table 1 shows a comparison of the hourly pay of a private ambulance company EMT (fire department EMTs are paid as firefighters) with other occupations in the same metropolitan area in the latter half of 1979.[17] The EMT's wage is not much above the minimum wage level. Big Al, a moonlighting EMT, made this relevant observation:

For sure this job doesn't pay much. I do better working as an LPN [licensed practical nurse], and I get more than twice the LPN rate as a med tech [medical technologist] in the lab at Atlantic [Hospital]. They have these machines now that you program to do analysis of specimens in the lab. It's all automatic. I have more actual responsibility on me when I'm working as an LPN, and more than that when I'm on the ambulance. Isn't that a pisser? The more responsibility you have, the less you get paid.

It was not unusual for conversations in Station Two to center on the meaning of a supermarket cashier's earning twice as much as an emergency medical technician.

In spite of the fact that people from higher social strata are now training as EMTs, it is still clearly a low-status occupation. It brings the people who practice it little prestige or power or pay. Ambulance work is, to use the simplest distinction among occupations, blue-collar work, and it is well toward the bottom of the blue-collar range at that.

The Character of the Work

Capable people are attracted to ambulance work in spite of its disadvantages. The National Registry once tried to find out why in a survey of EMTs which asked each respondent whether he took up the work "because of the excitement," "to help my fellow human beings," or "to earn a living."[18] Since the prospects of earning a satisfactory living at this job are meagre, the main attraction must be to the character of the work itself, to the method ("excitement") or to the mission ("to help"). For some people these intangibles may adequately compensate for the low status of the work, at least for a while.

Several features of ambulance work distinguish it from other occupations. None of these characteristics is unique, though perhaps their combination in one job is singular. They might appeal either separately or in combination to people who would as a result prefer this kind of work.

To begin with, there is a *concreteness and immediacy* about the job that is not true of many occupations. A run can be understood as a complete unit of work requiring intense application of the worker for a limited time and producing a visible service. The EMT is able to recognize a beginning and an end to his performance and to have a sense of what it accomplishes, even though he rarely learns about the fate of his patients. This kind of activity stands in contrast to the fragmented operations of the assembly line, the ambiguity of administration, and the long-term outcomes of farming or teaching.

Second, and of great importance to several of the Liberty employees, the work is *not routine*. The demands and pace of the work cannot be precisely anticipated. Each day has its own number, variety, and arrangement of runs; each run differs in details from all others. Thus the workers are protected from the boredom of knowing what will happen. However, this protection may weaken with time. Though the work differs from moment to moment, the differences grow less significant to the practiced eye. What appears to new workers to be an ever-changing panorama of events may appear to the experienced worker to be simply more of what has gone before.

Third, because the demands of an emergency take precedence over social conventions, ambulance workers are granted a provisional *suspension of the rules*. Like other medical personnel, they are allowed to make intimate physical contacts and inquiries about personal matters that in different circumstances would be expressly forbidden. Beyond that, they are permitted to violate normal traffic rules and other formal restrictions. They enter places where they would ordinarily not be admitted—expensive restaurants, the working floors of factories, police lockups, private bedrooms. They disregard codes of etiquette (intruding into a funeral service), of privacy (entering restrooms of the opposite gender), and of formal authority (giving directions to personnel in city hall). These exceptions to everyday rules provide the personnel with a taste of freedom which, though temporary, is genuine. For a few moments the ambulance attendant is magically outside the limits of commonplace social regulations.

Fourth, since emergencies can occur in any location, ambulance workers have an *opportunity to explore the backstage* of social life. They see the hidden side of the familiar when they enter the unexpectedly barren rooms of a fancy house or the greasy kitchen of a fancy bar. They see what is generally unfamiliar when they are called to dilapidated tenements or seedy hotels, to the soaking pits of a tannery or the boiler room of a freighter. Perhaps even more striking and disturbing, they see people who are in a backstage mode, whose defenses are down, whose polite roles have been shattered by crisis. This kind of street work is always instructive and usually interesting, and thus is especially attractive to young people.

Fifth, the job enables workers to *display uncommon skills* insofar as they are able to cope with situations others consider frightening, disgusting, or mystifying. The more unnerving a situation is to us—and most medical emergencies are unnerving—the more credit we are willing to give to those who can handle it calmly. The person who can deal with blood, pain, distorted bodies, and the various discharges of sickness is somehow special. Experience alone allows the ambulance worker to appear cool; what is shocking to the public is routine to the initiated.[19] Thus the EMT can often sense the appreciation and even the respect of those who call upon him, and feel satisfied at having been of genuine service.

Sixth, however marginally, the ambulance worker is able to *participate in the mystery of medicine*. He knows what is at the end of the hospital alley behind the big, red emergency sign. He becomes acquainted with physiology and anatomy, the meaning of vital signs, and medical terminology. He learns the importance of symptoms, the effects of drugs, and the recommended emergency treatment for specific conditions. He shares gossip with the medical staffs and hears about disagreements among doctors and the failures of medical care. He considers himself an insider in the allied health professions and might claim the right to a share of the prestige accorded the medical establishment.

In formal terms ambulance workers are included in the U.S. Census Bureau category "Service Workers, Except Private Household." Within that listing they are described as "Health Service Workers" and more specifically as "Nursing Aides, Orderlies, and Attendants." The latter category included 751,983 employed persons in 1970. This service worker classification is not in itself very useful. It includes detectives and dental assistants, busboys and bootblacks, and thus encompasses occupations of widely different kinds and various skill levels.[20] Table 4-2, which presents material from several sources combined into a typology of occupational characteristics,[21] provides us with a better instrument for examining ambulance work. A comparison of different kinds of occupations reveals two more characteristics of ambulance work that might attract capable people.

In Table 4-2 professional work is taken as the standard and the other types are constructed in terms of the degree to which they resemble the professions. This approach is in accord with popular thought in that "professional" is widely used to mean adhering to the highest work standards, and many occupations aspire to be called professions. As a consequence of this approach, however, actual professionals closely fit the characteristics of their type, while other occupations only approximately fit theirs. The EMT most nearly matches the "skilled" category, with two important exceptions—degree of supervision and nature of commitment.

The ambulance worker in the field is necessarily *free from close supervision*. To some extent the crews can manipulate the situation to give themselves greater control over the conditions of their work by not clearing promptly, by claiming a need to service the rig, or by defining a run to the dispatcher as more complicated than it really is. But even when their procedures are unexceptionable, the basic-life-support EMTs operate with a minimum of direction. (In contrast paramedics, the advanced-life-support EMTs, must consult higher authorities before initiating most procedures.) They do not differ from other skilled occupations in making routine field decisions, such as choosing a route or selecting a backboard, stretcher, or stair-chair to carry the patient to the car. Sheet metal workers, for example, make decisions on the basis of general principles to deal with the unique aspects of each job. Ambulance attendants do differ from most other occupations insofar as their own determinations directly affect the health and well-being of another person. The EMTs decide, for instance, whether to discourage a person from taking the ambulance, whether the patient should be treated for shock, whether they should run hot to the hospital, or whether they should initiate cardiopulmonary resuscitation.[22] Together the lonely responsibility and the potential seriousness of such decisions resemble the professions more than typical skilled occupations.

Professionals have a large measure of autonomy in their work because of the mandate they receive from society to supervise matters in their area of expertise. EMTs mimic the professional condition through what Eliot

Table 4-2
A TYPOLOGY OF
OCCUPATIONAL CHARACTERISTICS

Types of Work

Characteristics of Work	Professional	Semiprofessional	Skilled	Semiskilled/ Unskilled
Basis of expertise	Knowledge of general theory	Knowledge of application of segment of theory	Practical experience in applying segment of theory	Experience in specific task
Training	7–10 years beyond high school	4–6 years beyond high school	1–2 years beyond high school	Brief on-the-job instruction
Transferability of skills	Licensure; monopoly of interpretation of theory	Licensure; monopoly of certain tasks	Certification; unionization; monopoly of certain tasks	Unionization; informal recognition of experience
Latitude in definition of work	Mandate to define own and others' missions	Define tasks related to assigned mission	Define operations related to assigned tasks	Assigned operations; often repeat same motions
Degree of supervision	Professional autonomy; supervise others	Bureaucratic controls; supervise others	Constant loose supervision	Constant close supervision
Control over pace of work	Determine schedule	Arrange tasks within schedule	Determine rate of effort within task schedule	Standardized, fast, steady rate of work
Nature of commitment	Ideal of service	Career; institution	Craft; livelihood	Livelihood
Examples	Lawyer Physician Clergyman	Nurse Social worker Librarian Teacher	Artist Carpenter Computer programmer Plumber Electrician	Sales clerk Longshoreman Machine tender Secretary Teamster

Freidson calls "autonomy by default."[23] Most workers are subject to fairly close controls because their superiors can get near them. Ambulance attendants in action are simply not accessible. They are like the policemen in squad cars described by Jack Olsen: "[The watch commanders] made their speeches and the troops drove off and did as they pleased: a block from the station they were King Shit again."[24] It is also true that the medical professions continue to consider ambulance work a minor ancillary activity and thus not deserving of great attention. This means that from the perspective of the health care system, the controls that are not possible are not necessary anyway.

Ambulance workers are like most professionals (and semiprofessional nurses and teachers, for example) in that they have an opportunity for *commitment to the ideal of service*. That is, their work can become more to them than a living or even a satisfying craft; they can regard it as a valuable contribution to the community. Certainly there are EMTs who do not have this feeling, but the fact that the majority of ambulance attendants are volunteers is strong evidence that among them dedication to service is high. There is evidence of this commitment among paid attendants as well. Most of them serve on ambulances in spite of meager rewards and even though alternatives are open to them. They show pride in their positions by displaying EMT insignias on their clothes and cars. They seek knowledge about their occupation in publications, organizations, and training programs. Many of them are interested in a career in some aspect of health care.[25] The clearest indication of their commitment, however, is the workers' involvement in emergency medical care off the job. At least 60 percent of the Liberty employees are active in volunteer services with fire departments, with rescue squads, with first aid units at rock concerts and fairs, or in teaching CPR or other aspects of EMS.[26] This involvement is costly to the EMTs in both time and money.[27]

These two characteristics of the work, together with those that approximate the skilled classification, are the basis for describing the EMTs as blue-collar professionals. (The literature and the oral comments of officials within the occupation use the term "professional" in self-descriptions and exhort the EMTs as professionals to strive for a better quality of service.) Because of the occupation's low status, the peculiar conditions of the work are probably its main attraction for those who enter it. It is thus important to recognize that some of these characteristics may lose their appeal in time. Lack of routine, suspension of the rules, and an opportunity to explore the backstage become less important as they become more familiar. Insofar as these characteristics are only temporarily rewarding, the disadvantages of the occupation will begin to take on proportionately greater weight with experienced employees. This may be part of the explanation for the rapid turnover in ambulance work.

Learning the Trade

Although EMTs are in a position to prevent permanent disability and even to forestall death, they can be said to receive minimal training. Yet the seeming incongruity in this is more apparent than real. (Perhaps the greater illogic is that they should receive minimal pay.) Since the techniques of basic life support are relatively simple, the fundamentals can be taught with but modest effort. Further, though EMT training may be called minimal, it is neither frivolous nor perfunctory. Under the guidance of the U.S. Department of Transportation and with the help of the American Academy of Orthopaedic Surgeons, an efficient design for a standardized EMT course has been developed and employed.[28]

The standard course comprises about eighty-one hours of class work, which includes lectures, films, demonstrations, question and answer sessions, practice of hands-on techniques, quizzes and examinations, and ten hours of clinical experience (usually in an emergency room). In addition, each trainee is supposed to spend three times the class hours studying the text and reviewing lecture notes. The course provides a rudimentary understanding of medical terminology, anatomy, physiology, and the meaning of specific symptoms and vital signs. It concludes with an examination of both theoretical knowledge and practical skills. Although many courses are of high quality, the training process in operation does not exactly mirror the official design.

Formal Instruction

The programs vary with regard to who takes the training, who provides the instruction, and what kind of learning is emphasized. Each of these variables can be a source of strain, and each is related to the auspices under which the training is carried out. In some states community colleges run EMT courses open to all students. Elsewhere enrollments are restricted to participants selected by public officials or course coordinators. In Metropolis a consortium of a private medical school, the county medical society, and a public technical college oversees the training of EMTs. Available seats in the limited enrollment courses are distributed among municipal firefighters, rescue squad volunteers, and prospective employees of private ambulance companies by a consortium committee. Thus each trainee has to be sponsored.

While this restricted approach gives the authorities close control over the program, it also creates problems. Many people who think they are interested in emergency care cannot get into the courses, and a larger than necessary proportion of those who do get in would rather not be there. Firefighters, for example, may be forced in to meet department quotas, and volunteers may enter solely to satisfy legal requirements. The reluctance of these people affects the efficiency of training both by influencing the morale and ambition of the classes and by increasing the rate of dropouts. The approach also limits the pool of qualified persons available to the private companies and causes them to hire people they might not otherwise consider.

The auspices under which the program is operated determine to some extent whether most of the instruction will come from physicians, EMS personnel, or others.[29] Each, while offering something valuable, also introduces particular difficulties. The physician's problem is in determining how much groundwork to lay down in explaining specific treatments. It is easy to be too meticulous, as this item from a lecture on the mechanics of circulation suggests: "There are 14 grams of hemoglobin for every 100 grams of blood; there is 1/2 ounce of hemoglobin in 1/10 of a pint of blood." Such information provokes complaints among the trainees during coffee breaks. "They're talking right over our heads. They're talking to other doctors." "We can't possibly remember all this stuff. How are we supposed to get ready for the tests?" "What does this have to do with EMT work?" A possible explanation for these inappropriate offerings is that many of the medical lecturers are volunteers whose knowledge about the course and whose preparations for it are accordingly limited. One of the coordinators pointed out that physicians like to use the photographic slide set prepared for the course because it reminds them of what they are supposed to talk about; it becomes a graphic lecture outline. The coordinator of one of the Metropolis programs, a paramedic, summarized his feelings about physician instructors: "Doctors are not much help in teaching the EMT course. They don't add much to the information we have from other sources; they are usually too detailed and too easily distracted; and almost none of them have field experience." Physicians seem to be more appreciated by the students in EMS continuing education programs, who are more knowledgeable than the starting trainees.

When the EMS regulations were new, many courses were coordinated (and probably some still are) by persons who had neither field experience nor medical expertise—registered nurses, educators, health care administrators, even volunteer agency officials. In these cases complications arise when instruction is by default left to the coordinator—not an infrequent occurrence.

Nurse James admitted she didn't know much about splinting. She got the knot for the traction sling wrong; she tied it a different way each time she demonstrated it. "I hoped Dr. Ong would supervise this, but it never seems to work out. . . ." She couldn't get the ambu bag to work on a manikin. She doesn't know whether a contraction of the diaphragm causes inhalation or exhalation, has never ridden in an ambulance, and doesn't think she'd have the courage to do mouth-to-mouth resuscitation.[30]

It is the practical sessions—where one is to learn the techniques of splinting, bandaging, CPR, taking vital signs, handling equipment—that suffer most from the coordinator's lack of experience, because textbooks and slides are not adequate substitutes for guided physical exercises. Without adequate supervision, the trainees are forced to pool their information and misinformation and muddle through.

Where experienced EMTs (usually paramedics) are the course instructors, there is a greater emphasis on matters of practical concern to the ambulance attendant. The paramedics, however, may give simple answers and ignore important complexities, pass on their own biases too readily, and be unable to answer background questions on medical matters. Curiously, practice sessions under paramedics are sometimes as disorganized as those led by others.

Whatever the auspices, the trainees have a deeply pragmatic motive. Their interest in learning skills emerges in a ubiquitous tension between book learning and practical experience. This division was bluntly expressed by a ten-year veteran of a police rescue squad, who was required to take an EMT course:

First aid and common sense is all it is. You don't need to know all the medical stuff we're getting here. Some of these people wouldn't even know what to do if they really had to treat someone. You get called out to an automobile accident and you never know what you'll find. Maybe it will be nothing much, but maybe it will be a real mess. We have a person in our unit at Redcliff who just glances at the book and passes the tests, but he doesn't know what to do at the scene of an accident.

This speaker was himself having great difficulty managing the book work. His situation and his statement are typical of many ambulance personnel who developed their skills on the job and whose knowledge is recognized frequently by instructors who excuse them from the clinical sessions of the courses. Though they have served on ambulances for years, have been licensed by the state (perhaps under a "grandfather" clause), and have reason to feel they have been doing good work, many of them cannot pass the Registry examinations. Three of Liberty's most able EMTs were in this position. Their problems seemed to be a combination of anxiety, disinterest, laziness, and misfortune rather than a lack of talent. For example, one of the crew chiefs, who was dedicated to and fairly well read in EMS, failed the CPR section of the exam several times. Since he was able to continue working anyway as a state licensee, he was disinclined to invest much time or energy in satisfying the Registry requirements. The tension between book-based and participation-based competence should ease as the proportion of previously experienced people in the EMT classes declines.

The trainees who have not had experience on an ambulance express their pragmatic interest in a different way. They are less concerned about determining the relevance of class work than about simply getting through it. They are interested in what kind of test is coming up, when it is scheduled, what it will cover, and whether they are responsible for particular medical terms. They grumble about test scores, the wording of questions, and why specific answers were marked wrong.

Garfield, whom Nurse James mistakenly but persistently calls Garfinkel, was complaining that he studied the books thoroughly but that the tests don't correspond to them. He is dismayed by the amount of material to be mastered. He even questions the fairness of the tests. Nurse James replies, "No one gets 100 percent on these tests because you know how multiple choice questions are. These are simply the best answers of those given."

This attitude is evident in their restlessness when the presentations repeat material (busy work), include too much material (system overload), or deal with material marginal to the tests or EMT work (enrichment). Class reactions vary from dozing off to whispering and subdued laughter to mutterings of "break" and wisecracks to loud groans to tossing gum and candy around. If no new information is likely to be presented, the trainees rarely stay around after the main presentation to improve their technical skills. Often the coordinators encourage the trainees to be test-oriented, and thus encourage their pragmatic inclination, by offering the tip that the next exam will ask several questions about poisons or that the last state exam was heavy on diabetes or that they should memorize the anatomical chart on page 41. It is, after all, to the credit of the coordinator if the students do well on the examinations.

One of the contributions of the formal course is to shape attitudes toward EMT work. The trainees hear repeatedly that the prehospital phase of emergency care is of critical importance. They also become more familiar, and it is hoped less uncomfortable, with the messy side of medical work by seeing films and doing clinical observations on childbirth, for example. While they might not develop the detached concern that is seen as a necessary part of physicians' and nurses' training, at times their emotional distance from the subject matter of their study is striking.

There was a triple irony at tonight's session on the respiratory system. One of the smokers in the class said loudly (and seriously) to another,

"Save your cigarette pack for me, will you? We're collecting them to get an iron lung for Coloda County."

The lack of awareness that one's occupational concern might have a personal application is not unusual; carpenters often live in dilapidated houses, plumbers have leaky faucets, and lawyers are found to be breaking laws. A recent article showed that among the students at a school of dentistry, seniors, though they had had three more years of intensive training, had worse oral hygiene than did freshmen.[31]

Apart from specific information and skills, the most important product of the course for the EMTs is a set of *decision rules.* These are informal norms drilled into the trainees so they can act without deliberation in an emergency.[32] Because most of the rules are informal they, and the emphasis put on them, vary from one course to another. Probably the most general rule is that the EMT should always treat the worst possible diagnosis. For example, where head, neck, or back is involved in a serious trauma, assume there is a spine injury—move the patient with traction, immobilize and transport him on a backboard.[33] A rule giving more specific directions is the ABC of emergency care: treat in order, Airway, Breathing, Circulation. Exceptions to the rules emerge as the trainees gain experience, but the rules continue to be the foundation on which the rest of emergency practice is built.

Getting Your Patch

The most visible sign of an EMT's qualifications is the colorful shoulder patch that shows he or she has been certified either by a particular state or by the National Registry of EMTs. Completion of the course of formal instruction is essential for getting the patch, but it is not sufficient. The requirements, which vary from state to state, usually also include passing a distinct set of standardized examinations, both written and practical. The National Registry has its own standardized examinations and in addition requires each candidate to have six months of experience working on an ambulance.

These certification standards are intended to insure an acceptable level of competence in practicing EMTs, but there are problems in applying them consistently and accurately. First, the emphasis and even the content of the formal courses vary somewhat. EMTs who trained in different places can be heard arguing, for example, about the merits and demerits of taping an airway in place or of using an oral screw—a device for opening the clamped jaws of a patient. As a result, the standardized examinations may favor some trainees and put others at a disadvantage. The testers also vary somewhat; in one examination the fact that half the testees failed the problem on long-bone fracture was explained by the instructors as due to the peculiar standards of one evaluator.

Second, there are difficulties in monitoring the examinations. Driven by desperation and granted an opportunity, some of the trainees are ready and willing to subvert the testing procedures.

Carol Jean Hipp said there was gross cheating in the back of the room where she was during the last test. O'Dell was asking her for answers. Some others were asking other people for help and several were boldly looking things up in their books. Later, when we had exchanged papers for scoring, Railles was bugging me to change some of the answers on his paper.

This passage from my research notes refers to one of the frequent mid-course tests. Classroom behavior was more closely controlled for the course finals.

Third, the coordinators "help" their students by making them test-wise, even though they want to maintain the integrity of the exams. One of the Metropolis coordinators told me:

You can get an idea of what my tests are like by looking at last year's final, but I don't allow any of the exams to leave this office. The answers tend to get circulated so I can't use the questions . . . . I don't believe in grading on a curve. If the highest person in the class gets 80 out of 100, that doesn't rate an A; the person was wrong 20 percent of the time. I want to be sure the person who treats me in an emergency does it right.

Still, the coordinators give their classes broad hints about what will be stressed on the written examinations.[34] Some people receive tips about how to impress the evaluators.

After lunch as I was going back to the assembly room for the practical, I met one of the other trainees in the parking lot. Though it was a very hot day he was putting on a long-sleeved shirt. "This way," he said, "they can't tell if your elbows are bent when you're doing CPR. Little things like that can get you failed."

It is in this practical section that the exam's integrity can be most easily compromised. Here the trainee is asked to respond competently to a simulated emergency. For example, someone will pretend to have a dislocated shoulder and a fractured femur; the trainees must assess the "victim" and stabilize him with the available equipment within a limited time. The specifics of these practical problems are determined by state or national agencies but they are implemented by local personnel. The familiarity of the local EMS people and the trainees can bias the testing procedures. One of the Liberty EMTs, for example, had three relatives among the evaluators when she was examined. Trainees in another course were given detailed descriptions of the particular practical problems that would confront them in the National Registry exam. Further, instead of being randomly assigned partners, they were allowed to do the two-man problems with the students they had practiced with throughout their course.

These conditions raise questions about both the fairness and the effectiveness of the testing procedures. The examinations are not measuring trainees' performances uniformly insofar as local people have inside information or other advantages over outsiders. They are not measuring the ability to apply general knowledge to specific circumstances insofar as the trainees have been told, and even drilled in, the precise "emergencies" they will encounter. Under these conditions it is difficult for certified EMTs to have a realistic idea of their own competence. The noticeable difference between the formal and actual training and testing programs may be significant.

Joe, who has been a firefighter with Metropolis for a year and was with Riverview for several years before that, said most of the guys on the rescue squads probably have at least taken the EMT course at some time. "But some of them are no good at it. You have to wonder how they passed the course . . . . Everyone in the fire department ought to be trained in CPR. We've had some 'codes' and you should see some of these guys try to do compressions."

The experience requirement of the National Registry is something of a "Catch-22," a regulation whose conditions are separately reasonable but in combination contradictory.[35] In this case the candidate cannot be employed as an EMT until he is certified, but he cannot be certified until he has worked as an EMT for six months.[36] The impasse created by these conditions has been overcome in some instances simply by interpretation.

The Registry requirement of six months' experience is a Catch-22. I tell my people to simply state that they've had the experience; we consider anyone who has completed the course has had the experience. I think the National Registry accepts these interpretations by now as standard.

But course work and practical application in the field are not the same thing, and to treat them so defeats the ostensible purpose of the regulation—to insure that the certified have had field training. The National Registry provides another route out of the impasse, the granting of *provisional* registration to trainees who have passed the examinations. They may apply for full board certification after six months of experience.[37] State regulations, which are constantly being adjusted to maintain a pool of accredited personnel, sometimes provide for a kind of "cheater's permit," which allows a person with as little as ten hours of training, for example, to crew an ambulance with a registered EMT. Thus there is no single standard universally applied in the certification of EMTs. To discover the qualifications of an EMT, one must identify his shoulder patch and determine exactly what was required to earn it.

Recertification

Keeping one's patch is possibly more difficult than the original earning of it. National Registry now requires that an EMT be recertified every two years by presenting evidence of the completion of an approved refresher course, participation in authorized continuing education programs, and retraining in CPR. Some state licenses for ambulance attendants may be renewed without additional training, however.

The recertification regulations are an attempt to establish quality control within the occupation. They are important because no other form of evaluation of EMT work has been institutionalized. (It is important to note that the same criticism can be made about full medical specialties.)[38] Formal evaluations are so rare that trainees complain they never even learn what their mistakes were on the National Registry exams. Those ambulance attendants, usually in volunteer units, who follow up on the patients they have carried get some feedback on their handling of the cases, but the process is not regularized. In some places ambulance companies schedule formal critique sessions with medical personnel at local hospitals, but such arrangements are not widespread. The medical supervisor for Liberty, a physician who volunteered his services, attended occasional in-services and inquired, for example, about incomplete EMT report forms; his comments, however, were neither thorough nor directed at particular attendants. The company owners added little to this procedure. They might mention that St. Christopher's was complaining about poor reports or chide the employees about poor spelling: "Some people—most of them aren't here—don't know how to fucking spell. They make it up as they go along. Juneau Avenue is not J-u-n-o. It's 'seizure' not s-e-e-z-y-o-u-e-r. Come on, let's be professional about this." Careful periodic evaluations of EMT services seem to be exceptional.

On-the-Job Training

Book work and classroom practice are not a substitute for field experience. It is only under emergency conditions that certain requisites of the job become obvious to the trainee and the means for meeting them are of interest. In this training process the senior crewmen must add the role of instructor to their other responsibilities. While they may appreciate the prestige it gives them, the Liberty EMTs are not completely pleased with the situation, because the steady turnover of personnel means the demand is constant. Flash complained:

I seem to get to work with all the new people. It's a pain in the ass because I have to keep an eye on the back as well as do the driving. I don't mean it's always that bad. I know you'll ask if you get in trouble. But some of these people think they know it all. You have to watch them. I like to drive but not for thirty-two hours straight. You need to tech for a while to get a break.

Now and then an experienced attendant will rhapsodize about the sheer pleasure of working with another senior person, about the beauty and economy of their coordinated movements when each person knows exactly what to do.

The new recruits receive three kinds of instruction: setting-specific information, general occupational skills, and advice on giving a convincing role performance. Each kind contributes to the total work behavior of the EMT, and each is necessary for the successful completion of assigned tasks.

Every work setting has its peculiarities. The EMT must invest considerable energy in gathering *setting-specific information,* even though it cannot be transferred to another work place. Examples of this kind of information are the geography of the service area, the layout of report forms and billing slips used by the employer, the location of stored equipment in the ambulances, and the differences in bell tones of the telephones. It is even necessary to learn the eccentricities of standardized instruments. The company's heart monitor occasionally discontinues its signal if it is jarred, a trait that disconcerts many an EMT who sees his patient's EKG readout suddenly go flat (indicating cardiac arrest). In heavy rain, water usually spills out of the overhead control panels in the ambulance cabs, drenching the clipboards that have been left on the "doghouse" (engine housing) and ruining the report forms. Of course coworkers also have their eccentricities. A few of the Liberty employees expect to use a precise routine for making up a cot. Others employ informal variations on the company ten-code; Barb and Oren use "10-71" to signal the driver that a fast, rough ride will not hurt the patient (usually a drunk), "so let's get rid of this turkey and get back to work."

On-the-job training also includes *general occupational skills* that can be applied in any setting. Some of these skills are nearly universal practices. The trainee learns how to attach the heart monitor ("white is right" means the white lead goes on the patient's right shoulder), how to "crack" an oxygen tank before connecting the pressure valve, and how to lift a loaded cot (knees bent, back straight, palms down on the lower bar).

Other practices that are handed down are matters of personal preference, tricks of the trade used by some EMTs but not all of them. The new attendant may hear from one of the crew chiefs that the velcro strap holding the resuscitation mask under the cot can be used to bind the wrists of a corpse, or that you should fold a quarter-inch of the tape under when you put it away so you will not have to search for the end when you are in a hurry, or that you "back up" someone who is backing down stairs with a stretcher by gripping his belt at the rear and leaning with gentle pressure against his waist. These tips are likely to be offered in connection with an assignment when their relevance is clear. Sometimes new personnel will seek advice from senior crewmen after the event.

We took a young woman out of the security building to County Hospital. She was lying on the floor of the cell block, diaphoretic [sweating], and complaining of abdominal pains. In the ambulance she started to gag and I got an emesis pan under her chin just before she threw up. I wiped her face with a towel but I didn't want to set the pan down where it would slop over the floor. So I handed it to the deputy sheriff riding in back with us; he held it gingerly the rest of the way to County . . . . [A couple of days later] I asked Jardine what you do with a full emesis pan when you're on a run. He told me to put it in the step well of the side door. If it slops over it will be out of the way and you can clean it up later by just opening the doors and turning the hose on it. He couldn't resist warning that I shouldn't step in it if I had to go out the side.

Though these practices might not be covered in textbooks, they are not arbitrary. They are effective, they have been tested by time, and they are important enough to have been passed down along informal communication networks from one generation of workers to another.

A successful role performance depends upon one's looking the part. Sociologists refer to this aspect of human behavior as *impression management*.[39] Whether it is done naively or for specific reasons, rookies are advised about how they can look like competent EMTs.

The most obvious forms of impression management are those consciously designed to influence clients favorably. Neat uniforms and clean ambulances are examples of these forms. The company's road cot is to be made up in a particular way—bottom sheet, smooth and taut, top sheet, Chux (absorbent pad), and towel folded in order under the pillow; blanket folded in the center of the cot, hemmed edge toward the foot; straps buckled snugly, one across the pillow, one across the blanket. Beyond that, some of the crews work out drills whereby they can drape a patient with a flourish; they spread the sheet with one fluid motion and unfold the blanket with a noticeable snap. They get some satisfaction from putting on a show of brisk efficiency, but their joking about it afterward is a clue that they do not take it too seriously. The new employee is advised, "Don't refold the towel in the hospital; people don't like to see them reused. Be sure to get the Chux with the absorbent side up, otherwise the urine will just run off onto the cot." The senior people have an interest in encouraging good work, because anything that enhances the reputation of the company will at the same time boost their own status.

In other respects the interest of the EMTs in conveying a favorable impression is even more obvious. In particular they want to be thought of by their peers and by the public as capable. It is the exceptional crew chief who will yell at his partner during a run. The more typical commitment to maintaining a good front is reflected in a statement by Jardine:

I never correct my partners in front of a patient. I may give them some advice. A little hint maybe. But I always make it sound like a suggestion. I might give them hell after we finish the run, but I don't want to embarrass them or upset the patient.

Here the impression management is thought of as being for the good of the patient—to avoid agitation. By watching others perform, the new EMT learns to make the right moves to convey an image of cool proficiency. He uses a flashlight to test the reactivity of a patient's pupils, even though the brightness of the room may render the reflex undetectable. His pen flies over the checklist on the report form, recording judgments about patient characteristics without hesitation. And when he is confident there is no medical need, he takes a set of vitals to create the appearance of a technically informed opinion before advising the patient to forego an ambulance ride.

An apparently common practice along this line is the EMT's concealment of his failure to detect one of the patient's vital signs. For example, if he fails to get a blood pressure reading, he learns to deflate the BP cuff but leave it in place on the pretext of wanting to take a comparative reading in a few minutes. Then he is able to make a second attempt without revealing that he missed on the first one.

The occasions for applying such deceptions are frequent in ambulance work. To some extent they may be due to attendants not having had, or not getting, enough practice to sharpen their skills. However, many of the failures are explained by the conditions under which the work must be carried out. It may be fairly simple in a well-lighted and heated hospital room to bare a patient's arm, position the BP cuff, locate an artery, and register the blood pressure reading. It is more difficult in dark, noisy, or cramped quarters with the patient in an awkward position. It is especially problematic in the back of a moving ambulance, where the sound of the engine, the jarring of the stethoscope and sphygmomanometer tubes, and the shifting of the patient's body all work against a clear reading. Most of the experienced EMTs say they never try to get a BP when the ambulance is moving; at most they palpate the artery to get an estimate rather than try to hear through a stethoscope. It should not be hard to appreciate the occasional indefiniteness of patient assessment in the field, considering that from time to time under better conditions patients are, for example, mistakenly pronounced dead.[40] Further, because ambulance patients are often in serious condition, it is not unusual for their vital signs to be so weak that it is almost impossible to detect a pulse or respirations. The breathing of some patients is so shallow it does not even fog the inside of a transparent oxygen mask. The EMTs learn to deal with these uncertainties by using other clues in monitoring the patient (eye movements, reflexes, throat sounds) and by using approximations or evasions in their reports.[41] In most cases the deceptions have no bearing on the quality of patient care but are employed simply to avoid embarrassment.

A large part of the attendant's impression management is for the benefit of EMTs and related service personnel. They try to conceal from each other their failures at those simple tasks by which their competence can be measured. Many claim, for example, that they never miss getting a blood pressure. Ironically, some of these claimants have suggested how such an incident could be covered up. Moreover, there are stories in the company folklore that reveal the ambiguities of patient assessment.

Jardine told us a story about Louie in the back with a failing patient. Halfway to the hospital Louie yells, "Hey, I don't think this guy has a pulse." Jardine says, "Whatta you mean you don't think he has one?" Louie says, "I mean I can't find one." Jardine says, "Well, maybe you oughtta start compressions." Louie says, "Yeah," and goes to work and Jardine cuts in the lights and siren and puts the pedal down.

The shared understanding that these uncertainties are inherent in ambulance work is part of what Hughes has called "guilty knowledge"—the recognition among its practitioners that an occupation routinely includes deviant attitudes and behavior, limitations, and even failures that are kept secret from outsiders.[42]

One of the means of impression management is the attendants' dress. The company sets a limit of two patches on the uniform smock (overblouse): the Liberty logo over the left breast pocket and one other patch (either National Registry or a state emblem) on the left shoulder. However, the attendants have more freedom to express themselves in the gear they carry. Nearly all the experienced EMTs have equipment holsters loaded with a variety of lights, forceps, scissors, bite sticks, knives, wrenches, and keys. Some have their own stethoscopes. The newer employees seem inclined to tote as little apparatus as possible, yet they, like their senior colleagues, develop *pocket rituals*. They put the same items into the same pockets each time they dress for work, even though they might not have an opportunity to use a particular item for months. Everyone carries a ballpoint pen; nearly everyone has a penlight; each includes his own medley of items chosen from an array of bite sticks, ammonia capsules, Tempodots, four-by-fours (bandages), alcohol wipes, safety pins, and other materials. These items are treated as an essential part of the attendant's personal kit, even though they are all available in the ambulance trauma box. The personal kits seem almost to serve as talismans, symbolic objects that offer protection and security in the face of the day's uncertainties.

The experienced EMTs occasionally inform the rookies about other implements that might be useful. Jardine recommends work gloves, like the scruffy, red pair he uses, to avoid being contaminated by messy cases, particularly neglected corpses. He also carries an eighteen-inch steel flashlight wrapped with black tape, which he finds handy for protection when he is forced to enter perilous regions.

The EMT who wants to impress people with his skill and style has to beware of being labelled a "hot dog." A hot dog is an enthusiast with no class, a show-off with no sense of when he is offensive or overbearing, a know-it-all who always has a different and better answer, an achiever who takes himself completely seriously. One of the attendants for another private company is a prime specimen of this type. He has three patches in addition to the company logo on his shirt, wears a heavy pistol belt with two equipment holsters and a flapped pouch, and carries a pair of handcuffs (presumably for violent patients) dangling from his waist behind. The Liberty crews raise a few chuckles by wondering, for example, whether he has considered filling his ammunition loops with ammonia capsules.

The kind of impression management I have described here is part of nearly any job. Further, ambulance attendants, like other workers, must perform for more than one constituency. They can be described as occupying a *role set,* an array of variations on the role of EMT, which they play for different audiences.[43] In this chapter we have looked at some of the ways in which the EMT is influenced by his coworkers—through his identification with the occupation, through his participation in formal instruction programs, and through on-the-job training. Next we will look at the employer, whose influence on the attendant is clearly seen in such workaday necessities as ten-codes and paperwork.

5

ten-codes and paperwork

The Organization of an Ambulance Company

IMPORTANT NOTICE

THE MANAGEMENT REGRETS THAT IT HAS COME TO THEIR ATTENTION THAT EMPLOYEES DYING ON THE JOB ARE FAILING TO FALL DOWN.

THIS PRACTICE MUST STOP AS IT BECOMES IMPOSSIBLE TO DISTINGUISH BETWEEN DEATH AND THE NATURAL MOVEMENT OF THE STAFF.

ANY EMPLOYEES FOUND DEAD IN AN UPRIGHT POSITION WILL BE DROPPED FROM THE PAYROLL IMMEDIATELY.

—Item on the bulletin board in Station 2

The EMT's view of himself as a "professional" has an important effect on his behavior. The formal training, the occupational literature, the shoulder patch, the association with coworkers, all support a particular occupational identity. If that were the only or even the dominant influence, we could expect all EMTs to act in a similar, textbook fashion. However, the actual practice of ambulance work does not take place in a textbook world. It takes place in a situation where resources are limited and where the practical concerns of the employer may conflict with the EMT's idea of what is proper.

In this case we will look closely at how a private operation, which we have called the Liberty Ambulance Company, structures the work of its employees. Similar constraints will affect any ambulance service, whether it acts under the auspices of a fire department, a police department, a city health program, a hospital, a volunteer agency, or another organization. Whoever has legal responsibility for the service will also have the authority to lay down regulations, directives, procedures, and suggestions that shape the workers' activity.

On the Job

When the ambulance attendant puts his skills to work, when he reports for duty, he does so not only as an EMT but also as an "employee" insofar as he is serving under the auspices of some organization. These two aspects of the role of ambulance attendant—EMT and employee—are sometimes mutually reinforcing, sometimes in conflict. Moreover, the relation between the two alters as conditions change. We can learn a great deal about such changes by looking at the experience of a new attendant who is getting on-the-job training as an EMT and at the same time learning what is expected of him as an employee. This experience can be described in terms of several distinct stages of development of craft and commitment.

Alone in the Back

At some point the driver slams the doors of the ambulance shut and the new EMT is for the first time alone in the back with a patient. No longer can he enjoy the observer's immunity from responsibility or hide behind the clipboard while a third man handles the direct care. At this point the EMT begins to understand the practical requirements of the job.

The patient is the tech's primary focus. That damaged human being in front of him is the one important variable in the rig's familiar compartment and the chief reason for the existence of an EMS system. The tech's attention is drawn especially sharply to the more critical patient whose breathing is labored or shallow, whose eyes are glazed and staring, whose complexion is sallow, or who is not responsive to word or touch. The life of such a patient seems unbearably fragile, as though the slightest neglect would allow it to flicker out. And the tech becomes vividly aware of how little he can do to forestall that event. He pleads silently that the patient last a while longer, and sometimes he voices these pleas as a kind of desperate treatment.

The visiting nurse was clearly alarmed by the condition in which she had found the old man. His complexion was pale and he was not responsive. B.Z. did get a reflex when he ran a forceps across the soles of the man's feet. The man's wife, who herself had a heart condition, rode to the hospital with us. In the ambulance B.Z. called back, "Get a good seat; we'll be doing a ten-seventeen." Gundy, the tech, was not sure we should be using the siren, considering the woman's bad heart. He was also worried that the patient's breathing was so low and that he was not responding. He asked the wife how to say "open your eyes" in Spanish, but he couldn't get it right. All the way to the hospital Gundy kept rubbing the old man's cheek and chanting a few phrases as though they would hold his attention and keep him alive—"Hey, Julio, qué pasa? Hang in there, Julio. You with me, señor? Julio? Hey, man, qué pasa?"

Out of experiences of this sort comes the incentive to employ more substantial treatments, such as cot adjustments, cold packs, suctioning, oxygen, and antishock trousers.

First, however, the tech must find out how to operate the equipment used in these treatments. It has suddenly become important to him to know that the suctioning unit works only when the ambulance engine is decelerating and that the different rigs have different valves for the oxygen, and different switch settings for the lights and air, and peculiarities like a loose rear step or a seat belt with a stripped anchor bolt.[1] Some potentially important facts are ignored because they seem to have no immediate relevance to patient care; few remember that the recorder for the heart monitor is in a black case under the squad bench, and fewer would be able to hook it up if they did remember. Other conditions that are relevant come to light only by chance. No one was aware, for example, that the lug wrench in Car 31 did not fit the wheel nuts until a crew had a flat during a run and had to call for a back-up because they could not change the tire. The tech's altered circumstances give a higher priority to such details, which earlier seemed to be of little consequence.

Being alone in the back seems to be a stimulus for accelerated learning. Information that was not part of the formal training program is now seen as valuable and is picked up quickly. For instance, because the tech must copy the data for assignments the crew receives while in the ambulance, understanding the radio is necessary. But to the newcomer, radio transmissions are mottly mumbles and static. By paying attention, however, he can soon recognize patterns of exchange—the dispatcher's lead mnd the crew's response—and even the tone and mannerisms of particular voices. Then he realizes that radio traffic has little content beyond numbers: ten codes, squad designations, times, addresses, and call signs. As the codes and the protocol of the transmissions become familiar, he is able to distinguish and understand phrases like, "Thirty-two is ten-twenty-three at County." It takes a bit longer to master the street names and the designation of squads in the service area. But eventually the EMT becomes so adept that he can follow radio scanner broadcasts subconsciously. When someone asks, "Where'd [Rescue] Unit Ten call from?", he can reply, "They're at a fire on North Fourteenth." This knowledge can be translated rather directly into response time and thus into the quality of care given to patients.

But while the patient may be number one, the tech has other responsibilities as well. There are also records required by the EMS system and by the company. Much of this information pertains to the patient's condition while in the ambulance, so the tech must learn to write on the run, a skill that requires practice and perhaps even talent, and to establish routines of patient handling that will allow time to fill out forms. In the earliest stages of the EMT's career it is the patient who gets the attention at the cost of the reports. The company is willing to grant the tech leeway while he is becoming acquainted with procedures, but soon it expects the paperwork to be properly handled.

Detached Concern

It takes only a few runs, perhaps only a dozen, to change the EMT's outlook. By the end of a week of full-time duty, the patients no longer make the dramatic impression they did at first.

As we walked to the bank parking lot just after midnight, Jase asked, "Have the patients begun to blur together for you yet?" Flash said, "Yeah, can you still remember all of them?" I told them I had asked Tanner around noon whether he could remember our second run of the shift. He said he couldn't. Neither could I.

This blurring phenomenon, which is recognized by the EMTs as a marker along the course of their careers, does not necessarily mean they have become less concerned about their patients. It does mean that the techs are more detached emotionally and more likely to see their patients as types of cases to be treated with routine courtesy.[2] Even so, while they do not follow up on their patients, as volunteers who make fewer runs might, the crews do remember. Occasionally one will scan the obituary columns and recognize the name of a critical patient he once carried.

This detached concern is a result both of the tech's becoming seasoned and of a refocusing of his attention. As the tech encounters conditions and cases that are repetitious, he alters his definition of what is significant. The third encounter with urine-soaked bedclothes may be as offensive as the first, but it is not as noteworthy; the third instance of diabetic coma is as serious as the first but not as alarming. It seems appropriate to speak of a working EMT as being "blooded" in the same sense as a combat recruit undergoing his baptism of fire. Without the moderating influence of controlled conditions or support staff (common to other health occupations), the EMT is quickly introduced to sagging flesh, stringy muscles, deformed toes and feet, unexpected growths, strange spots, odd calluses, rotten teeth, swollen joints, rashes, scales, bruises, and wrinkles; he becomes accustomed to the sight and smell of strangers' sweat, spit, urine, vomit, blood, feces, and pus. The disagreeable features of patient handling, which are something of a shock to all rookies, continue to be a subject of conversation for veterans but less as a source of dismay than as a nuisance to be cleverly managed. As these features become familiar to the new tech, the individuals who possess them become less distinguishable.

While the tech is finding the patients slightly less engrossing, he begins to get feedback about his handling of the paperwork. The balance of his attention shifts somewhat in the direction of the latter. The Liberty crew chiefs, responding to questions or making spot checks, point out insufficiencies in a rookie's reports. Nor is it unusual for the owners to telephone the new EMT during his first week with a suggestion about how to make their lives pleasanter by being more careful, pointing out that the ambulance service is intended to be a profit-making enterprise. Thereafter, criticism about illegible writing, misspellings, inconsistencies in names or addresses, and incomplete information is communicated in notes from the office staff or directly by the owners in company meetings. The owners want precise reports so they can bill their customers, as well as protect themselves from possible legal action.[3] The crews want the office personnel occasionally to ride the cars as observers so they will appreciate the difficulties of producing neat, accurate, and thorough paperwork in the field.

The paperwork demands are nicely symbolized by the digital clock on the ambulance dash; it produces new data steadily, and the tech must refer to it for the times of notification, dispatch, response, arrival, departure, delivery, and clearing. It takes a while for those necessary glances at the clock to become habitual. The company holds the tech responsible for four forms on each run: the bill or trip slip, an EMT report, a Medicare form (if appropriate), and a release form for the patient's insurance company. Three of these require signatures plus an assortment of license numbers and policy numbers (for Medicare, Medicaid, or an insurance company), phone numbers, zip codes, and addresses (for the patient, the next of kin, and any employers). In addition, certain cases call for "prescription" forms from a nursing home or "incapacitation papers" from the police department. Runs outside the county involve the calculation of an extra charge for mileage. The forms have different layouts, are of different sizes, and have carbons attached. It takes a great deal of manipulation to fill them out on a steady table top, let alone having to deal with the irregular motion of a vehicle. Further, the tech feels the pressure of time. The forms are supposed to be filled out before signatures are requested (a rule that is rarely observed), and the EMT report is to be handed in at the hospital before the crew clears. (While the police and the rescue units also have to process a lot of paper, they are relieved of the bother of billing their customers and collecting signatures, and they can postpone completing their reports until they are in the station after their runs.)

It is safe to say that any of the allied health occupations would claim that quality patient care is their primary goal. It is also safe to assume that the self-interest of the workers and of their organizations determines how their priorities are put into practice. In ambulance work there is a conflict of priorities when paperwork competes with patient care for the tech's attention. The tech is under considerable pressure to collect and record information at the scene and on the way to the hospital just when the patient might need to be closely monitored. This conflict was perhaps most apparent when the company added a new form to the set for which the EMT is responsible; there was of course no increase in the time available to the tech for filling it out.

The EMTs are very much aware of the situation. Jilly exclaimed more than once, "I take care of the patient first, period! The hell with the paperwork!"[4] The patient is in the company's hands for less than an hour, but the trip slips and the EMT reports are in process and in the files for a long time, not only within the company but also in the hospitals, now and then in the office of the medical advisor, and on occasion even in the courts. In this conflict the EMT's reports serve both sides; if the paperwork is not done, the EMT has no evidence that the patient's condition left no time for the paperwork![5]

These increasing demands help to weaken the new tech's preoccupation with the patient. To be sure, some of the paperwork (the EMT report) might effectively channel the tech's concern to specific symptoms. But the

rest diverts his consideration from the medical aspects of the case to matters of immediate importance only to the company.[6] It probably takes three
weeks to a month for the tech to get the paperwork under control.

Obsession

As the tech realizes he can cope with the demands of ambulance work, the
job begins to dominate his life. Some attendants, even when they are off
duty, notice every siren. Some, like Louie, arrive at Station 2 as much as
an hour before they have to go on duty. Some talk about the job too
much; Sonya's friends asked her if she thinks about anything other than
the ambulance. This combination of continuing anxiety and growing confidence seems to produce a feeling close to exhilaration. Jilly expressed it
this way:

*I just love working on the cars. It's like a drug; once you start you can't
stay away from it. After I've been off for sixteen hours I begin to get
restless. . . . Here even the routine isn't routine, if you see what I
mean. You can live half a lifetime in half an hour on a good call.*

Having overcome the fear of working one-on-one with ailing patients and
having managed the burden of paperwork, the rookie begins to feel less
like an imposter and more like a genuine EMT. This new attitude is apparent in the tech's eagerness to improve his performance, in his ability to see
the humor in his ineptness, in his adoption of crew slang, and in his cata-
loguing of new experiences.

The obsessed EMT avidly collects advice on routine matters, such as
dealing with the paperwork, positioning the adjustable road cot, and doing
a two-man lift. And he is less likely than before to feel threatened if the
learning is somewhat at his own expense.

*[On Sunday afternoon] Jase and I were running hot on Spring Street to
the Rivereast apartment district. Suddenly I felt a burning sensation
on the left side of my abdomen. I muttered something like "Damn!
What the hell is this?" Jase yells over the siren, "What's the matter?" I
yell back, "I don't know. It feels like I'm on fire." He shouts, "Are you
all right?" I am looking for smoke by now but instead I discover a wet
spot under the seatbelt. Then I reach into my smock and pull out the
remains of an ammonia capsule. Jase sees it and starts laughing.
"That's why I never carry those in my side pocket," he hoots. I smiled
a little.*

The crew slang becomes a natural part of the new tech's seeing and saying. He uses the accepted shorthand language—"Do you remember our ten-twenty-three on that last run?" He makes accurate distinctions between concepts, realizing, for example, that the crews use "the core" to mean not the downtown area of the city but the black section to the west of it. He becomes less self-conscious about using informal codes, such as "ten-sixty-nine," which is a label for cruising the main streets to look at the scenery (particularly women). He might even slip it into an official call, as in "Thirty-one to dispatch. We're ten-eight and ten-twenty-four. Request a ten-sixty-nine along the boulevard."

The obsession also emerges in "collecting firsts," which refers to the common practice of rookies letting the others know when they have handled specific problems for the first time.[7] Among the firsts the crews notice are certain patients—the puker, the Rescue Mission referral, the belligerent drunk, the backboard extrication, the psycho, the shock victim, the DOE (corpse), the emergency childbirth, and the pulseless nonbreather (requiring CPR). Other firsts are associated with particular places (Gino's Bar or the stadium) or particular circumstances (a major blizzard). The veterans sometimes use these firsts to remind the rookie of his inferior status ("So you don't know about Gino's, eh?" or "You mean you've never been on a 'baby call'?"). Further, because the new techs are uneasy about the landmark events they have not yet encountered, the veterans rag the rookies by trotting out stories of their own firsts to increase this uneasiness. Many of the stories are part of the crew culture and have been polished by retelling. They are performed in a kind of ritual, with each senior EMT taking the floor in turn and describing his own version of a first experience. The following story of a first DOE is typical.

It was a slow night. About as bad as this. Bachman, the shithead, was on the phones [dispatching] so you know things couldn't be going too well. We were all half asleep except The Doctor, and he was completely asleep. Shithead calls with a "head-to" [start driving toward a possible call] for 3300 Sweeter, so I wake The Doctor. He is annoyed. "You gotta be kidding. That's only ten blocks from here." [Little to gain by leaving early.] But we cruise down and see a paramedic rig and a police car and a crowd on the lawn. The Doctor says, "Damn, I'll bet it's a DOE." About that time the shithead gets on the radio and makes it official: "Respond ten-seventeen for the Fire Department. . . ." We pull up in front. Our response time is about eight seconds. One of the mobiles [paramedics] comes out and says it's a DOE about a day old. The Doctor says we won't transport if it's too bad, and he calls dispatch. I get all brave and go to take a look. It's completely dark so I have to feel my way around to the back. There's another crowd in the back yard; I don't know where they come from. I go up *the steps and some people on the first landing tell me it's another flight up, naturally. The electricity is off, so I'm creeping up these narrow stairs with my penlight. It's like Halloween. At the top of the stairs I turn toward the doorway and Bam! there's a face on the floor just inside the room. It looks kinda normal, except the eyes are half closed and nothing is moving. Across the room a couple of cops are going through the guy's wallet with a flashlight. About then The Doctor stumbles in and we assess our patient. He's a big mother. Looks like Ernest Borgnine. He's not as stiff as I expected, but he's lying in a puddle of something with his feet under the sink. We set up the cot downstairs and bring in the rubber gloves and the rest of the crap. The portable light is about as bright as two matches. We decide to go with the folding stretcher since the scoop [stretcher] might pinch enough to cause him to purge. We get the guy strapped and covered. The Doctor took his end down first and got most of the weight. I may look stupid but I knew I didn't want to be on the bottom if that guy's bowels let go. The stairs were a bitch, naturally. The weirdos were still out there in the gloom getting their rocks off looking at a corpse. On the way to County I checked out his wallet, which the cops turned over to me. There was an alien registration—from Poland—some other cards, a folded piece of paper, and a Social Security check for over $200. No cash; I guess the police were protecting that! The paper was about twenty years old and said the guy was "King of the Over World, in Secret." Those were the exact words. There was a bunch of other shit about his entering the country and some signatures. You couldn't tell what it was all about, but it was strange. I took a look in the back and the blanket was starting to work off the guy's face. My hair stood up. I'm not kidding you. We pissed away about a half hour at County just waiting for one of the interns to get off his ass, walk over, and pronounce the guy. When we finally uncovered him under those bright lights, he looked a whole lot worse than he did in the dark. His face was bluish-purple. When the intern felt for a carotid [pulse], some fluid came out of the guy's nose and ran down his face. The Doctor said it was about the worst DOE he had seen in two years with Liberty. He said if he had got a good look we wouldn't have transported. Did we go over that rig! We washed that fucker right there in the parking lot with water, alcohol wipes, disinfectant, and anything else we could slop, splash, or spray. The run took two hours by the time we finished. It was just a coincidence that we cleared at midnight [when the shift ended].*

The period of obsession is a honeymoon in the relationship between the new tech and his company. He is fresh and enthusiastic and feels a pride in his work place as well as in his work. He is eager to please and readily ac-

cepts suggestions for improving his performance. Thus the company finds
him easy to socialize to its procedures. The new tech does not yet have a
basis for critically evaluating the operations of his company, nor is he willing to accept the sometimes cynical comments of the senior EMTs. The initial emphasis on the ideal of patient care and the subsequent emphasis on
the organization's requirements are for a time in balance. The period lasts
for about three to six months, while the new tech, gradually becoming
aware of his own career interests, attempts to make a place for himself and
to move up within the company.

Making a Place

At some point the tech realizes he is no longer simply a rookie. The realiza-
tion may be triggered by another EMT chatting with him about "the new
man," or by his being paired with a freshly promoted crew chief who needs
the support of a seasoned tech. Other attendants begin to think of him as a
"regular," as one who is OK, who can be depended upon not to lose his
cool during a run. He has caught onto the crew routines, both formal (re-
supplying the rigs) and informal (setting the siren on manual at switch-off).
And he has learned to manage the personal details of his work, such as
handling contact lenses and laced boots when he sleeps in quarters (wear
glasses and sleep with your boots on). He may even display his new sense
of security by testing the limits, perhaps by having a cigarette in the ambulance cab under the NO SMOKING sign.

The EMT must make a place for himself both among his fellow workers
within the crew society and as an employee within the company. The two
social networks are related but not identical. The crews are primarily concerned about attitude and personality, the company about dependability.
At Liberty Schaeffer was considered the front office's "golden boy" but was
not a favorite of the crews; Gundy was well liked by his fellow workers but
was fired for being unreliable. Whether the new employee is aware of it or
not, he will fit in only if he is able to satisfy the distinct demands of both social groups.

It may take a few weeks or a few months to achieve the feeling of being
part of the operation. Some people never quite fit in. Others seem to belong from the beginning. Among the factors that determine how quickly an
EMT feels comfortable on the job are his technical skills and attitude toward ambulance work, his personality, and certain social characteristics,
such as age, race, and gender.

The most tangible evidence that one is a member of the crew society is
the key to Station 2. Each employee shares in the mutual trust implied by
the valuables left in quarters. But fitting into the crew society is not simply a
matter of having access to the physical environment. It is primarily a prod-

uct of the positive and negative sanctions employed by the crews. One of the simplest indicators of positive regard is the nickname given to a new employee. Based on first impressions, these nicknames—The Doctor, Crash, Miss Liberty—show that the employee is recognized as an individual.[8] However, the nickname can as easily be used in derision as in comradeship. Good-natured teasing in public, private sharing of confidences, and invitations for beer and pizza after the shift are more significant indicators of acceptance. When someone does not quite fit, the crews use a variety of negative sanctions to change his attitude or behavior.

The crews communicate their feelings about particular attendants through jokes, advice, and overt criticism. Jokes are often vehicles for serious concern about sloppy data, slow paperwork, skipped station duties, reckless driving, or smelly socks. Advice is a direct attempt to help someone who might not realize there is a problem, but it implies that one of the EMTs is superior to the other. Overt criticism is a last resort. It sometimes ends in a shouting match, though it is not necessarily motivated by hostility; B.Z. and Lyle, both highly skilled EMTs, can at times be furious with each other yet soon forget their rage and be eager to crew together. If none of these approaches improves the culprit's behavior and if the feeling about him is nearly unanimous, he goes on the "shit list"—an informal roster of employees who are the butts of gossip and jokes when they are not around and who may become negative legends after they leave the company. People who make the list are complainers, goof-offs, incompetents, and hot dogs. It is clear to all the other attendants who is on this list—for example, Blaszkiewicz, Schaeffer, Bachman, van Buskirk—but because those listed seem to be insensitive to public opinion, they might not be aware of their position.

A specific case will illustrate the process by which the crews exercise social control over their individual members. Blaszkiewicz, who constantly and futilely works on his hair, was quickly nicknamed "Brush." He was welcomed as new blood, and because he had worked for Liberty in the old days, his outspokenness was accepted as a legitimate expression of his long experience. Within a week, however, the reading on Brush changed from bright prospect to dull pain. He complained about everything, bothered any females within reach, sulked when he was corrected, and let his uniform become wrinkled and dirty. Nor did the quality of his work compensate for his bad attitude. He was poor at relating to the patients, his reports were inaccurate and often illegible, and on one occasion he went to sleep in the back during a baby call. As these problems emerged, the crews tried to get Brush into line by joking ("Hey, Brush, you're supposed to write this stuff in English, not Polish. Can *you* tell what this says?") Because he seemed to miss the point, they made more direct approaches ("Brush, Harold wants to know why we don't have ten-twenty-threes on any of this morning's reports. What do I tell him?") When that failed, the crew chiefs setting up the next shift would let him overhear that no one wanted to work with him ("Fuck no! I put up with his shit all day Monday. I'm working with Dandy today.") Brush became more sullen and more negligent, and the crew chiefs became more hostile; eventually they complained to the owners. Finally, when the chiefs flatly refused to work with Brush, Harold got him to apologize and to promise to shape up and got one of the senior EMTs to agree to work with him for a trial period. After two days that arrangement fell apart, and in exasperation Harold fired Brush. The story of the firing was big news around quarters for a week.

When the crews are concerned about an attendant's competence it has as much to do with aptitude as with formal qualifications. They distinguish between "street" EMTs and "gerrie-work" EMTs. Street EMTs have the stuff to deal with emergency situations in the field—the technical knowledge, the practical ability, and the inclination. Gerrie-work EMTs are only reliable for moving bodies and for dealing with patients (usually geriatic) who are not very responsive.[9] Brush was judged to lack the stuff ever to be a street EMT, which Liberty's work required, and because of his careless paperwork was not even good with gerrie work.

The new EMT must also make a place within the company's formal structure. The ambulance company, like other organizations, is concerned about both producing something customers, contributors, or taxpayers are willing to buy, and maintaining enough internal order so work will be efficient and agreeable. The Liberty owners judge an attendant's production by the quality of his paperwork and by his reliability, and judge his disposition by reports about his attitude and by evidence of how he follows rules.[10] Those who are sloppy (Blaszkiewicz) or who too often fail to show up for work (Gundy) are dropped on the first count, and those who cannot get along with other attendants (Bachman) or who openly violate regulations (Jase) are dropped on the second. In special cases complaints from outside may get an attendant fired even though he is satisfactory in other respects. Emergency room complaints about his flippant attitude contributed to the firing of van Buskirk.

Even attendants who are otherwise in good standing with the owners can work themselves out of favor by blatantly ignoring regulations. Jase, as we have already seen, was a dedicated and competent EMT. Unfortunately he could not restrain himself from playing with the radio.

Flash says Jase is one of the biggest abusers of the radio. He told me he called him the other day when Car 32 wouldn't start and said, "Jase, I need you to jump me." Jase replied on the air, "I'm not into sex this week." Soon after this a notice went up on the refrigerator in Station 2: "RADIOS ARE FOR BUSINESS ONLY."

He used the radio to talk with his girlfriend when she was dispatching. Some of the EMTs thought Jase's playfulness was cute, but others considered it childish. Eventually the violations were forced to the owners' attention.

Harold was testing the radios because the signals had been breaking up and asked for a five-count. Jase called back with "One, two, . . . , . . . , five. How was that?" Another time, when Harold was synchronizing the dispatcher's and the car clocks, he asked Pete by radio, "What does your clock say?" Before Pete could reply, Jase cut in with "Tick-tock, tick-tock."

This casualness about company regulations, augmented by a growing depression and disenchantment with ambulance work, led to Jase's eventual departure.

Social characteristics are also important in determining whether an EMT can make a place for himself in a company. Liberty is staffed almost totally by young, white males, but older and nonwhite men can fit in with a little strain. Racism is tempered as people get to know each other, though it never disappears completely; racial slogans are heard in quarters if there are no blacks present. Flash probably expressed the view of most of the attendants when he cursed upon seeing a black man strolling hand in hand with a white woman. "I'm prejudiced. I'll admit it. I still can't get used to seeing that. But then you meet someone like Gundy and you can't help but like him. He's a good guy." Female attendants face a similar difficulty and, since there are more qualified women than nonwhites looking for ambulance jobs at the moment, sexism is probably a bigger problem than racism in the companies. Women feel the simultaneous effects of cultural inertia, sexual rivalry, and gender status.

People are most comfortable acting in familiar ways. In social institutions that have been dominated by males, familiar means men talking to men, often about women. Male dominance has been as pronounced in health care institutions as in other sectors of society.[11] Most women entering ambulance work encounter an exclusively male orientation. This male orientation is offensive, on the one hand, because it draws unwarranted distinctions between the genders (This is not women's work.) and, on the other hand, because it ignores legitimate concerns of females (What difference does it make that there aren't any women instructors?). This male orientation is partly the result of a conscious "stud" philosophy that values females mainly as sexual objects, and partly a thoughtless continuation of trite jokes and expressions, an example of what we might call *cultural inertia*.

The stud outlook is obvious in the girlie magazines in quarters and in the whistles and wolf calls of firefighters in the field. The male orientation carried by cultural inertia is more pervasive and more subtle. It turns up in the best places. For example, when one of the most respected and well-liked emergency medicine physicians led a seminar on gynecological and obstetrical injuries (a specifically female subject), his presentation included a great many male-oriented phrases:

You look at your girl and. . . .
Your mother gets ready for Thanksgiving and then. . . .
I don't understand women's hormones myself. You all know how to
  make a hormone, don't you? You don't pay her!
What a man would recognize as a trapped fart. . . .
Your wife ever do that to you? They start. . . .
I decided to go into the diseases of female genitals a little because I
  thought you'd like the dirty pictures.
You sometimes run into these guys. They suffer from lack-of-nookie
  disease.

Although a sizable minority of his audience was female, none of the physician's remarks recognized a clearly female perspective. (Nor were any of the seminar's other leaders female.) At most he suggested that our perspectives affect our behavior and that these perspectives can be faulty. His demonstration of this point was a further expression of the male orientation.

Let's go, men. We're going to have a demonstration of rape. I need
some volunteers. All right! Look at that response! Now this is going to
be a male-male sexual assault . . . Where did they all go? See, you
guys immediately assumed rape involves women. Not true.

The male orientation is usually reinforced by innocently humorous sexual references, because this humor, whether introduced by men or women, seems to focus on the female.

Some of the men were smiling and snickering when Nurse James was
instructing us on how to deal with a prolapsed cord in emergency
childbirth and said, "That's the only time you should put your fingers
into the vagina." She herself giggled.

The results of cultural inertia in EMS are seen at the top of the authority structure as well as in formal training and at the level of day-to-day operations. A prominent physician insults a fellow member of the County Council on Emergency Medical Services in a public meeting, because although she is "only" a nurse, she has challenged (legitimately) one of his opinions. A physician (male) lecturing on shock points out that the femoral (thigh) artery is not good for checking a pulse because it looks bad to pull up the skirt of a fallen woman. And male-oriented jokes become a natural part of in-service training sessions in the company:

HAROLD: *How many of you have opened the OB (emergency child-birth) kit?*
ATTENDANT: *You mean the one on the shelf or the one on the cot?* (General laughter.)
HAROLD: *We're losing our decorum.*

Another barrier to women easily making a place in a company is the *sexual rivalry* they occasion among the males. The romantic or sexual possibilities of relationships increase their emotional intensity. In quarters horseplay (like pillow fights), teasing, and even debating about where to eat take on a special flavor when they occur between men and women. When women workers are in short supply, an undercurrent of jealousy and competition among the men emerges in episodes of showing off and in mild antagonism. Speculation about attendant romances is prevalent. For example, Oren and Barb spent a lot of time together. They worked the same shifts, almost always crewed together, and often would come to work in the same car. They even developed the same skin rash, though Barb claimed it was a kind that spread without contact. Barb had a boyfriend named Leon who, while he sometimes called her at Station 2, was never actually seen by the crews. A popular theory was that Leon was really Oren trying to disguise his voice as part of a scheme they had devised to keep their relationship secret. The elusive Leon protected Barb from being hassled by other males and protected her and Oren from being hassled by the company. The mystery of the relationship was never cleared up, but the two were seen driving together after both had quit the company. While they worked at Liberty they were treated as though they were romantically paired. Sexual rivalry is obvious only as long as the women are unattached or otherwise available.[12] Once the women are understood to be committed, they are granted a more routine place in the crew society, though the men may still flirt with them.

Another hurdle women must cross in making a place in ambulance work is *gender status,* the understanding that gender is the primary basis for determining one's social value and societal role. The most familiar expression of gender status is the macho (super male) attitude. The macho attitude of male superiority is acted out in the field when firefighters try to be helpful by taking over the heavy work. Sonya was furious when one of them tried to take her end of the cot as the crew took a patient downstairs. "I don't give a damn how they feel," she said. "I'm getting paid for this job and I'll do it. They can keep their hands off unless I ask for help." The macho attitude also turns up in a blander form in the sentiments of males who do not try to project a he-man image.

Oren was trying to show he was broad-minded [no pun intended] about women working as EMTs. He said Slaterville, his hometown, has had women as volunteer firemen for a long time. "They are great for fighting brush fires when the men are away. And after a run, while the men are folding the hose, the women will go and start the food. Actually, one of the men is pretty big on cooking, too. I think he's the buyer."

The men support their gender status not only by affirming what they can do, but also by describing what women cannot do. Ambulance work, which requires considerable physical activity, provides opportunities to claim that men are better suited to the job. Since there have been relatively few female attendants, these claims are usually based on logic rather than experience. Because the claims are supported by knowledgeable people, they become part of the wisdom that is passed along to each new generation of workers and thus can be challenged only by dedicated individuals. Anderson, one of the coordinators of EMT training in Metropolis, supported the view of female inferiority.

Anderson said he wasn't bothered by the fact that women were prevented from becoming paramedics because they couldn't get into the fire department. He doubted that women could do the heavy work required. "A 140-pound woman simply doesn't have the upper body strength of a 140-pound man." As support, he cited one of the private companies: "The one Nagel has. I forget the name. Towner! He had two women working for him but now they don't make runs any more." Anderson said he would not want to be on a rig with a woman if they had a very heavy person to carry.

Both men and women are influenced by the opinions expressed in the classes (as well as by similar outside opinions), especially because they have little or no practical experience with which to counter them. This influence can be seen in a conversation that followed a training exercise in extricating patients from an automobile.

Mrs. Paroleck, a large woman, said, "I don't think women are strong enough to carry the heavy patients. I know I don't have much strength in my arms. I couldn't lift some of these big people." An experienced trainee (male) standing nearby agreed. "I've never seen a light patient to be transported. They're all heavy." Carol Jean Hipp thought two men and a woman would work as an ambulance team but not two women and a man. The policeman from the Redcliffe rescue squad pointed out that a call that involved a person who was violent as well as injured would make a difficult situation for a woman.

In fact women seem to do very well on the Liberty crews.[13] Heavy patients are not noticeably a problem for them. Of the three cases I was aware of when backup crews were sent to help with a lifting problem, two involved a female; in the first assistance would have been required even if two men had been on the scene, and in the second a woman was on the crew sent to help. Barb routinely does the necessary lifting, shares the driving (including running hot) with her partners, and is prepared to defend herself if a patient becomes unruly.[14] She admits to losing her composure only once on a run—when they were called to a pornographic bookstore. When circumstances unexpectedly required Sonya to drive the ambulance to a hospital, she managed it very well, even though she had had no experience. Jilly handled the carrying acceptably until she was injured in an accident that did not involve lifting. Because their performances are much the same, as the women gradually adopt the men's mannerisms, including swearing, about the only distinction between the genders in the loose-fitting uniforms is that the women wear their hair longer.

Those men who work directly with the women EMTs seem to get along with them best. The front office attitude toward them is not as clear. While the owners are willing to hire women and to treat them like the men, they contribute to the male gossip about women being moody or emotional—"What's the matter with you tonight; got the rag [sanitary napkin] on?" The owners do not question the women's competence but are inclined to accuse them of being egotistical or defensive if they stand up for what they consider their rights or interests, for example, Barb complaining about Oren assuming it is his prerogative to clear for them on the radio, or Sonya complaining that the station chiefs do not adequately supervise the checking of the rigs. The company seems to be concerned about romantic entanglements between men and women attendants, but not about male homosexual pairings, which are as possible and as potentially disruptive.[15] Moreover, a female attendant said an owner had once hinted that he expected sexual favors. The owners promoted Barb to crew chief but forced Jilly off the roster[16] and were happy to see Sonya leave.[17] Since the personalities of the women are pertinent to their evaluations, it is impossible to draw any conclusions about how sexism in itself affects the company's treatment of women.

Women are often ambivalent about their roles as workers. (Some of the men are ambivalent about their roles, too.) They are flattered by the whistles of the studs at the same time that they are offended by them. As the quotations above show, the women are not always sure they can handle the demands of the job. Even Barb admitted she was uncertain about whether she wanted to accept a promotion because she did not know if she was ready for the additional responsibility; she finally accepted it because she wanted the extra money. When the women are not confident about their abilities and aims, the uncertainty of the company about women workers is intensified, and it becomes more difficult for them to fit in.

Making a place, then, is not automatic. Nor is it simply a matter of technical competence. It requires adjustments on the part of everyone involved. Some people are less able than others to make, or to convince others to make, those necessary adjustments.

Moving Up

The EMT who becomes part of the company has met only minimum standards of acceptance. Most attendants are eager to have it recognized that their qualifications are more than minimal. They can achieve this recognition informally in competition with their peers, privately through increases in wages, or publicly through an advance in formal rank.

There is little evidence of serious competition among the attendants, but there are continuous minor skirmishes about their relative experience, skills, and accomplishments. Arguments about proper procedures, displays of such esoteric knowledge as how to set an IV by doing a "cut down," or exhibitions of such special competencies as interpreting EKG strips or repairing a radio are occasions on which an EMT can establish at least a temporary superiority over his fellows. A more visible and more practical way of moving up is to develop a proficiency in two specific areas—dispatching and driving.

The company is forced to use attendants as dispatchers because it is difficult to find and keep full-time people. Dispatching is boring, confining (often one cannot leave the radio even to go to the bathroom or to get a drink), and stressful (when too many calls or other complications arrive all at once). It pays even less than working on the cars. Moreover, full-time dispatchers are handy targets for criticism.[18] Clark issued this complaint about a dispatcher who had been on the job for several months (an unusually long time):

Alice is a nice lady but she's not a good dispatcher. You have to say everything twice because she never hears it the first time. She gets the squad numbers wrong. Sometimes you tell her you're en route to the hospital with a patient and she'll tell you you're 10-19 [return to quarters]. But she's better than these other two guys they just got! Can you believe it? They fuck up constantly. They lose track of the cars. They don't answer the radio; half our transmissions are "Dispatch, do you read me? Do you copy?" When they do answer, they mumble and you can hardly understand them. They don't even keep the [trip] log right. The next dispatcher has to catch up all the stuff from their shift.

In spite of the disadvantages of the work, some of the attendants are usually willing to fill in for a shift. It offers overtime pay, it is a change of pace from making runs, and it is an opportunity to perform for the rest of the crews. Proper dispatching requires knowledge, intelligence, and discipline. The dispatcher has to sort through a jumble of noises—the scanner brings in all the fire department traffic, the radio brings reports from company cars, and several telephone lines bring routine and emergency calls. He must know the service area well enough to locate scenes quickly; he must know the status of his crews at all times; and he must know whether to deal with a particular call by paging a crew, sitting on it, or giving it to another company. The EMTs differ in their inclination to take on this extra duty and in their ability to cope with it. The one who handles it with efficiency and flair is respected; the one who never quite masters it (like Bachman) continually reminds the crews of his deficiencies.

Another skill the EMTs develop through experience rather than formal training is driving hot. Because the vans handle differently than most automobiles, new attendants begin by driving them back to quarters to get the feel and to practice using the side mirrors rather than the rearview. Driving hot does not come naturally, and even after six months the experienced Louie was reluctant to do it. Jase, who sometimes works as a flying instructor, advises learners to drive at first as they ordinarily would except under lights and siren; they can increase their speed as it feels comfortable.[19] Moreover, driving hot is not simply guiding a high-speed vehicle; it is also picking the best route and proceeding without hesitation. Driving hot is, like dispatching, an accomplishment that draws a clear distinction between attendants.

The company tries to improve the general skills of its attendants by posting notices, sponsoring continuing education programs, and offering in-service training. These efforts not only promote professionalism, they also have the practical consequences of advancing the employees toward recertification, satisfying public (and municipal agencies') expectations, and presumably creating group solidarity. Notices, posted on the bulletin board, included in the handbook updates, and announced at company meetings, usually concern equipment and work procedures. These communications are effective for the full-time people, but part-timers, like The Doctor, complain that it is usually a month before they hear about new regulations. Assessing the impact of the other approaches is even more problematic. When the company offered to cover their expenses at a local day-long seminar, less than one-sixth of the attendants showed up.[20] When the company organized monthly in-service sessions, only 25 to 55 percent of the employees attended, in spite of the promise of refreshments and bonuses toward the purchase of uniforms for attenders and vague threats against nonattenders.[21] The low participation rate is not due solely to the EMTs' lack of free time; a competing private company, CityMed, had higher attendance rates at its in-services. Last-minute planning, haphazard publicity, and uneven presentations undercut Liberty's efforts.

The company takes such achievements as driving, dispatching, and attending in-services into account in determining pay rates, though people receive small increases on the basis of experience alone. Still, the pay of even the most experienced tech is less than that of a crew chief.

Officially, moving up in the company means becoming a crew chief. Although there are a station chief, a supervisor, and a director of in-service training, these positions are essentially small additional duties given to the most senior attendants and likely to be altered periodically. Crew chief is a stable position superior to that of other attendants in responsibility, authority, and pay. Like sergeants in the army, the chiefs are valued for their experience; they know "epistaxis" means nosebleed. In the field they interpret company policy on cleanup, paperwork, head-tos, drunks, criteria for shock, speeding, use of oxygen and solid expendables, taking certain supplies inside in cold weather, and everything else. Because the chiefs may differ in their interpretations, the tech adapts to the chief on his own crew. The owners, from their side, expect the chiefs to have the company's interest at heart in avoiding overcalls, hurrying when there is a shortage of cars, and trying to collect for services on the spot when possible.

Crew chiefs are also the company's primary means of quality control. First, they represent a rank which itself provides an incentive for good work. (When this incentive was threatened by an experienced but newly hired EMT who was advanced to crew chief after only three days on the job, the attendants were outraged, and the other chiefs complained that he did not even know the company procedures. The three-day wonder stayed on and made a place for himself, however.) Second, the chiefs serve as company agents for socializing new employees in correct practices through on-the-job training. Third, while the owners also receive comments from outside sources, get feedback at in-service meetings, and note the thoroughness of the billing information, they rely most heavily on the formal and informal reports of the crew chiefs as a way to monitor the attendants' activities.

Liberty, following what seemed to be the predominant pattern in medical services until recently, did not have an established technique for periodically evaluating performances. Therefore it did not verify how well its method of quality control was working. It appeared that over time the chiefs became lax about checking out the rigs, for example, when there was a crew change, but such impressions can be misleading. The EMT reports, however, offer a more reliable basis for estimating the level of attendant performance.

One appropriate indicator of the quality of patient care is the record of vital signs on the reports. Checking vital signs—pulse, respirations, blood pressure—is a critical part of patient assessment which is emphasized in EMT training. The Liberty personnel agree that it is an essential practice: "Jase says you should do vitals even if the patient is only there because of some minor trauma. He says you don't want an apparently sound patient to fall over on you in shock." The medical advisor shows his support for the practice by inquiring about a report that is not complete. And the company sets the principle down unambiguously: "9.2Bd—You should record at least one full set of vital signs on every emergency call or emergency transfer call." Since nearly all of Liberty's runs are for these kinds of calls and since even some of the nonemergency transfers have to have their vitals monitored, the vast majority of the reports should include records of vitals.

A survey of all the completed EMT reports in the collection basket at Station 2 on eleven occasions over a six-month period showed that 59 percent did not record *any* vital signs.[22] Many reports listed only a single sign, and therefore less than 41 percent had a complete set of vitals. Even if one run in five was a routine transfer that did not require close monitoring, less than half the emergency patients were given a complete assessment. Table 5-1 shows that the crew performance apparently improved during the four sampled months. This could be evidence of a real trend, since the company was changing during this period: an increasing propor-

Table 5-1
COMPLETED EMT REPORTS
WITH ANY VITAL SIGNS RECORDED

Month	Number of Reports Checked	Number of Reports with Any Vital Signs Recorded	Percent with Any Vital Signs Recorded
May	62	11	18
June	80	27	34
July	30	12	40
October	154	85	55
Total	362	135	41

tion of attendants were National Registry-certified, the company tightened its organization by establishing supervisory positions and issuing a handbook, and feedback from local emergency rooms and from the medical advisor began to accumulate. However, it is not possible in this study to identify the separate contribution of each factor. Moreover, the apparent trend toward improvement may be a statistical accident, since it is less evident when we look at the figures for each survey occasion. Except for two occasions in May (when few reports included vital signs) and one in October (when many of the reports noted vital signs), the figures are nearly all in the 40 percent range.

When the EMTs are asked (by the owners or the medical advisor) why their reports are not complete, they give any of several explanations. First, there is no time to get vitals because of outside pressures—the police want the street reopened, or there are dangers from spilled gasoline or hostile bystanders, or the firefighters who offer to help carry a patient are in a hurry, or the company wants the car to clear as soon as possible. Second, there is no time because the hospital is only a minute or two away. Third, the patient may be uncooperative or even belligerent. Other explanations are less likely to be reported publicly but are mentioned in conversations in quarters. When the primary complaint is obvious and limited (for example, a young and healthy softball player twists her ankle during a game), it is awkward and embarrassing for the EMT to treat the injury as though it were a major trauma and act like a doctor. Sometimes the personal desires of the crew—they are hungry, they want to get out of the cold, the patient is filthy—tempt them to take shortcuts. Finally, confusion on the scene may hinder the crew from getting full information and force them to depart earlier than they would like, thus interfering with the recommended assessment. While these excuses are not considered legitimate according to the principles of EMS taught in formal courses, they take on a legitimacy from the practical experience of the attendants.

Liberty does not routinely use report data to monitor its crews, nor does the agency that oversees EMS for the state.[23] Rather the company depends on the crew chiefs to maintain acceptable levels of patient care, and the state depends on the company to regulate its employees.

The time required for an attendant to move up to crew chief varies. The EMT who made the jump in three days was considered an exception. Flash said he had "only" worked for a month when he was made a crew chief. Barb and Louie, on the other hand, worked for more than six months before they stepped up in rank.

Burnout

Few EMTs can realistically hope to make a career of ambulance work, and fewer can expect to make it with a private company. The attendant suffers from *blocked mobility:* his position is a dead end because it offers no opportunity to move in gradual steps up a ladder of occupational advancement.[24] Now and then a Liberty employee will move out or over—one used his volunteer firefighter status and a change of residence to qualify for a paramedic training program, and another got a job as an EMT in a hospital—but eventually most leave paid EMS work altogether. The new EMT is not particularly concerned about the limited opportunities, because the work is interesting, there are increments in pay and the chance to become a crew chief, there is the possibility that the company will expand and create new positions, and there is the dream that someday the city might open the paramedic ranks to nonfirefighters. However, within the first year, perhaps as the pinch of low wages increases with marriage or children, the limited future becomes obvious. The high hopes that supported dedication to the work turn into disappointment.[25] Attendants begin to say, "There's a limit to how long you can jockey an ambulance; you can't push a rig all your life."

While he is becoming aware of his meager prospects, the EMT might also begin to show the effects of the persistent stress of the job. Stress here refers to the emotional tension we experience as we try to meet expectations in moments of crisis, in hours of fatigue, and during long periods when we are repeatedly discouraged.[26] We see signs of stress when Sonya, at her first emergency childbirth, calls out, "Here comes the uterus," and when Tanner, at the end of a double shift, furiously swings the ambulance around corners until the top compartments unlatch and air splints and cervical collars spill into the back.[27] We see the results of continuous and enervating stress when, after a year on the job, the usually precise Lyle becomes blatantly careless. In prolonged periods of anxiety or in repeated instances of challenge the emotional arousal takes a toll on the spirit and body, its effects surfacing in outbursts of frustration and rage and depression and in physiological abnormalities.

Individuals vary not only in what they perceive as stressful, but also in their physiological responses to stressful stimuli.[28] Liberty employees blame the job for affecting, among other things, their metabolism, sleep, and blood pressure. Quite a few of them are overweight to the point of having a "spare tire" around the middle. Extra eating becomes a way to relieve boredom, a means of self-comfort, and finally a habit for them. Yet some of the biggest eaters do not gain weight, which suggests that they respond to the job by burning more energy. Louie, one of the slenderest EMTs, said he gained weight on vacation but lost it as soon as he came back to work. That the workers often look tired may simply be a consequence of the many shifts and the long hours they work, or it may be related to the irregular schedules or even to the impossibility of relaxing on the job. Lyle claimed he could not sleep around quarters because of the atmosphere. Jase said he took the job home with him and had nightmares about the worst cases. Several of the men have elevated blood pressures. Dick, a college student working for the summer (he could have made better money installing phones but found ambulance work more interesting), discovered he was showing the blood pressure of a person twice his age. He said that was not normal for him and attributed it to stress caused by the work. The Doctor failed a physical examination for the Coast Guard Reserve because of hypertension, which the physician considered serious. The Doctor said in the past his blood pressure always went down when he was not working.

There is reason, beyond the claims of the workers themselves, to think ambulance attendants have high-stress jobs. When occupations are ranked according to the degree of job stress, lower status health workers (licensed practical nurses, clinical lab technicians, nurses' aides, dental assistants, and health aides) are near the high end of the scale.[29] Ambulance attendants would be included in this broad category. Such lists, however, oversimplify because they ignore the great variation of conditions within each occupation and the specific factors that are related to stress.[30] A study sponsored by the National Institute of Occupational Safety and Health analyzed these factors more carefully. Eight of ten conditions listed as promoting high stress are characteristic of the job of the private EMT: fluctuation in workload, responsibility for the well-being of other persons, unpredictable task requirements, exposure to conflicting expectations, uncertainty of future career, underutilization of abilities, low pay relative to comparable occupations, and little participation in decisions about the organization of work. The study linked these conditions to job dissatisfaction, which in turn was linked to certain forms of illness.[31]

Most of the company attendants eventually become disenchanted with their work. For some the change is gradual.[32] Time away from the job helps them realize something is different. While a few days off might have them feeling slightly uneasy about returning, a vacation that allows them to "see how other people live" causes serious misgivings. Louie, who used to report an hour early, said that after his vacation he no longer looked forward to work; he hated to come in. For others the change seems more sudden and might even be traced to a specific event. Gundy was shaken when his crew was sent to pick up "the bionic drunk," a wild man with a switch strapped to his side and wires running under his coat to what he claimed was a bomb. Gundy soberly said, "I don't need that action." Jase was shaken by a big psycho, who was so frightening that Jase preferred to have an unprepared Sonya drive rather than allow her in the back where the guy threatened to jump out of the moving rig or to throw Jase out—"and he could have done it!" Shortly after this, a patient kicked Tanner in the head and sent him to the hospital, which dispirited Jase further.

As the attendants' attitudes change, so does their behavior. They look and act tired, they complain, they admit to being depressed, they are apathetic about their duties and indifferent toward their patients, and they speak cynically.[33] These are essentially the fatigue and distancing behaviors characteristic of the work-related physical and psychological exhaustion referred to as burnout.[34] The condition seems to be common in jobs that combine direct contact with clients, significant responsibility (life and death), uncertainty of outcome, and ambiguous authority—that of the intensive-care nurse, for example—but has been applied to a wide range of helping professions.[35] Although the effects of burnout are felt by the friends and family of the worker,[36] it is the job itself that gets the full impact. The condition so compromises the worker's effectiveness that programs have been established by employers to enable their people to prevent or cope with it.

Not all ambulance workers are victims of burnout. Some paramedics, usually employees of organizations with better benefits and job prospects than the private companies, stick with the job for a long time.[37] Even a few Liberty employees, like Tanner and B.Z., have maintained their enthusiasm and their jobs for several years, but they are exceptions. The situation is not likely to change because what appear to be the contributing causes of burnout—low pay, a limited future, role conflict—are not under the control of the company organization. They originate in the ambiguity of the place EMS occupies in the wider social structure. We will examine this subject in Chapters 7 and 8. Nor are the consequences of burnout, particularly the turnover of personnel, felt only by the company, they are also shared by the wider society.

Turnover

There is little to keep the private attendant on the job once he becomes disenchanted with the work. In other organizations accumulated retirement benefits and points toward advancement might hold the worker, but the private EMT lacks these incentives.[38] The dim prospects in ambulance work, together with more promising futures in other lines, result in a high rate of turnover. During the first two years in the Metropolitan EMS system, two-thirds of Liberty's attendants stayed less than a year. Because of this turnover, the company must invest resources in finding and orienting new attendants. Quality control safeguards are weakened because the crew chiefs are distracted and allowances are made for the new workers. While the company pays lower salaries to the less experienced, it may earn less because of fouled up paperwork, wasted supplies, and lost time.

The employees themselves feel the strain of turnover. The crew chiefs complain that they work harder because they must keep an eye on the new people. Everyone loses some of the pleasure of good work since there is little opportunity to develop smooth coordination with new people or to crew with experienced people. The desire to increase their skills declines as the employees realize there is little likelihood of occupational advancement.[39] Moreover, the morale of the crews is affected. They feel an implied rejection each time a familiar worker leaves, and perhaps a growing reluctance to invest much in getting to know his replacement. Eventually the senior attendants begin to look at the job (and talk about it) as a revolving door and to plan their own exits. They are not happy about their leaving, but they become resigned to its inevitability.

The turnover has consequences for the public, too. The effectiveness of the crews depends to a large extent on their experience in the field. If the ambulances are constantly staffed by new people, the patients do not receive the benefits of fully trained attendants. Whether an improvement in the level of care would be worth the cost is a matter to be debated by policymakers, but there seems to be little doubt that the loss of years of attendant experience makes a difference in what the public gets for the money it now pays.

The Union Episode

The EMTs are aware that their fates are affected by forces outside the company—the federal and state standards that allow local control, the county statutes that put the fire departments in charge, and the department policies that only firefighters may be paramedics. Still they try to make what gains they can by negotiating with the company. These exchanges usually concern such small matters as whether Station 2 should have a microwave oven or whether the TV should be serviced out of the employee fund. Once, however, in what was a shock to the owners and a sobering experience for the attendants, there was a movement to unionize.

Until that time Liberty had been a paternalistic enterprise. It began when, in a friendly fashion, the owners split off from CityMed over policy differences. The new business was nearly all transfer work, and the owners, Harold and Pete, worked the cars along with some of the people who were to become crew chiefs. There was little distinction between the crews and the front office; a feeling of being part of a common endeavor predominated.

A change in attitude followed Liberty's being given responsibility for one of the four sectors in the city's new EMS system. The number of calls, cars, and crews increased. The owners felt they needed more office space and moved into a six-room suite, but the crews were left to operate out of a women's lavatory ("The first rule is that you *never* use the toilets in this room!") in a temporarily vacant hospital building. The attendants felt cut off from the owners and began to talk about the lavish offices and the big profits the company was earning. The owners claimed they had a cash flow problem (the time lag between the filing of claims and the insurance payments) and big expenses, and that they were earnestly searching for suitable crew quarters with adequate parking. The EMTs began to voice complaints about low pay, poor working conditions, and even lack of job security. Meanwhile someone had the Teamsters union local drop off some cards formally requesting membership, and enough EMTs signed to force a vote. The owners first heard about it in an official letter from the Teamsters. They were furious because of the attendants' ingratitude, because of their manner of expressing it, and because the owners considered the Teamsters to be about the worst of the union locals. The attendants were mildly amused, hopeful, and apprehensive.

The company decided it would be too costly and too risky to contest the election by calling for a hearing. Nor did they follow the lead of other companies that had faced the same pressures: the owner of Towner reportedly challenged his employees to a fight in back of the garage; Wright fired the attendants who were trying to organize a union; and Safety Lift went out of business until the employees' union vote was no longer in effect. Instead, the Liberty owners tried to get a strong vote against Teamster representation. They talked privately with each employee, pointing out that the union would cost a considerable amount in dues, would reduce the flexibility in company regulations ("If someone missed a shift we would be forced to fire them"), and would destroy the cordial relations between the front office and the crews. They promised that as the cash flow problem eased, improved conditions would immediately follow and there would be a committee of employees to handle grievances. The company benefited from its reputation of being fair with its employees. Though the owners tried to "fish" in part-time attendants to avoid paying overtime, if a full-time employee was financially strapped, they would cut a part-timer's schedule to give the full-time person extra work. Even in a tight pinch Liberty did not offer moonlighting firefighters higher pay than their own regulars, as some companies did. Most important, the owners quickly found a location for Station 2, complete with kitchen, comfortable furniture, rug, TV, sleeping quarters, and study room.

The official election was by secret ballot. The attendants voted strongly against representation by the Teamsters.[40] All but a few of those who had earlier been strong supporters changed their minds by the time of the election. Thereafter, the situation seemed to get better for a while. The back room was indeed furnished with a desk as a study, but it soon became a part-time office and eventually a locked office and storage. A crew organization was established for cleaning, ordering supplies, and filling schedules—tasks formerly done in somewhat irregular fashion—by creating the new ranks of station chief and supervisor. The employees elected an advisory committee to consult with the owners. Unfortunately Harold was angry that the election was held without his knowledge and that the elected did not include one of the people he favored. The committee certainly did not operate as a supplementary organization to the formal authoritarian structure.[41] It helped work out a "last chance" for Blaszkiewicz, but little more was heard from it. The business continued to expand for a while, and Station 1 was constructed in another part of the sector to complement Station 2.

As the operation settled into a routine, the senior people began to complain about the company again. Jardine was disgusted that although the number of runs per shift was triple what it had been before Liberty joined the EMS system, the pay was as low as formerly. He vowed that he would no longer willingly do extra jobs, such as taking inventory. When Schaeffer quit and the owners were criticizing him after he was gone, the crews began to consider whether they might be bad-mouthed in the same way. When the three-day wonder was promoted to crew chief, they thought they noticed an arbitrariness in the front office. When Jilly was maneuvered out of a job, they talked about an appeal to the Labor Relations Board. But the attendants did not make any serious protest. The number of calls declined and stabilized. The company settled on the minimum number of cars it could run and still meet its responsibilities. And most of the senior EMTs drifted away to other jobs.

A reasonable interpretation of the union episode is that it provided at least a diversion and perhaps even a small hope of change for attendants who had begun to understand their dead-end position. Once they had given the matter more consideration, they realized that the union was not likely to improve things and might even make them worse. The post-election changes captured their attention for a while but did nothing to alter their pay rates or their career prospects. The company was not in itself the problem and could not by itself provide a solution.

Thus the employer organization affects the EMT's behavior both by what it does (enforcing regulations within a particular structure) and by what it cannot do (offer career advancement to positions outside the company). These effects are felt not only in the company's maintenance activities, but also in patient care. Together with the formal training program, the company organization accounts for a great deal of the EMT's handling of patients, but not all of it. The characteristics of the patients themselves also influence the EMT's behavior. Even nonmedical characteristics become important when the attendant begins to stereotype patients and to react to them in terms of such categories as shit calls, tunas, and tearaway ties.

shit calls, tunas, and tearaway ties

Crews and Their Clients

---

*"Come ride in my ambulance," the
paramedic said hospitably.*
   — a Tom Swifty by Pauline Gayle

From the idealized outlook of formal training, the EMT is taught to treat patients equally and solely on the basis of medical need. As an employee, the attendant receives a similar message with some additional directions about judging whether an ambulance conveyance is appropriate. In the field the influence of ideals and directives is diminished and sometimes obliterated by the attendant's reaction to the tangible patient. Each patient is more than a set of signs and symptoms; each attendant is more than an assessor and recorder of physiological functions. The individuals serving for the moment as patient and attendant are at the same time willful persons who react emotionally to each other. Patients vary as to social properties, personalities, and settings; attendants vary in their responses to these characteristics.

At 11:30 PM we got a call to the "Eggs Benny" luncheonette downtown at First and Spring. Alma_____, 71 yo w/f [a seventy-one-year-old white female], was sitting on the toilet in the tiny restroom. She claimed she couldn't get up. The manager, who wanted her out of there, said she probably had a heart attack. Alex went back to talk with her, Cliff made a big show of rolling his eyes while he got some information from the firefighters of Rescue Squad 18, and I went out to the rig and got the stair-chair, because it looked like we would have to carry her around some tight corners. We all gathered at the open restroom door, where Alex was trying to convince Alma to get up and use her walker. Cliff made a few soft-voice comments about being at the end of our shift; Alex told him to take it easy and back off. I pushed the stair-chair up next to the door, and Alex curtly told me to get it out of there. He resumed sweet-talking Alma off the toilet. Cliff was impatient and I was pissed at having been corrected. The squad left and Cliff said, "Eighteen doesn't know shit. That young guy doesn't have a clue about what's going on." About that time we heard a commotion behind us, and there was Alma shuffling along with her walker and Alex behind her smiling. No heart attack. He didn't give her a ride to the emergency room, just a little encouragement. He said she was worried about her weak knees. Cliff wrote, "No transport—No medical need" across the bottom of the trip slip, and we headed for the ambulance.

Confronted by Alma, three EMTs reacted in three different ways: one looked at the clock, one looked at the terrain, and one looked at the patient. The differences were not simply due to a division of labor. They reflected the different priorities of the EMTs in that situation, different ways of handling a particular patient—as an individual to be motivated, as a body to be moved, as an assignment to be completed. Possibly the priori-

ties went beyond that situation and revealed something about the personalities of the attendants. On an earlier run it was again Alex who had gently
talked with a sobbing teenager who had been attacked on the street in front
of her house. Although he had not been able to convince her to let us take
her to the Sexual Abuse Treatment Team, Alex calmed her and got her to
consider reporting the incident. Cliff and I would probably have had her
sign a release slip and left.

If Alma had been of another race, age, or social class, the reactions of
the crew might have been different. The attendants do adjust their behavior to the patient. Yet this great potential for variation in patient care not-
withstanding, EMT activity on most runs fits within a few recurrent and
predictable patterns. In spite of the individual proclivities of the crew members and occasional exceptions, broad categories of patients elicit similar
behaviors from the attendants. There seems to be a widespread agreement
among them about how patients should be classified and about how the
various classifications should be treated. In other words, the EMTs stereotype the patients and pass these attitudes along to trainees, with the result
that the stereotypes become institutionalized.[1] The tendency to stereotype
is supported by the EMT's lack of substantial background information on
the patient and by the necessarily brief and temporary relationship. In displaying this tendency, EMTs are no different from physicians, nurses, and
other health care providers.[2]

Some of the stereotypes express the kinds of demands the patients
make on the crews' talents. On good runs the patients give the EMTs an
opportunity to display their professional skills and to be on their best
behavior. The patients associated with three other broad categories—shit
calls, tunas, and tearaway ties—require that the attendants give their attention to other than medical concerns. Finally, there are a few rather specific
social categories of patients that get special recognition and treatment from
the EMTs.

Good Runs

EMTs frequently enter Station 2 announcing that they had a good run. In
this context "good" has at least two meanings. It means either that the
crew members were required to use their professional skills or that something interesting happened, or both. Of the two, a run that demands skill is
better than one that is merely interesting.

*B.Z. and Flash came in and said they'd just saved a life. They had a GI
bleeder [the patient was hemorrhaging internally] who had vomited
about a pint and a half of blood. She had a systolic blood pressure of*

65 and a rapid pulse. They got her out of her wheelchair, put on the MAST pants [Medical Anti-Shock Trousers], and elevated her feet. Her blood pressure came up immediately. They didn't inflate the pants but used them as a backup. They were afraid the added pressure would increase the rate of internal bleeding. They took her to Mercy [Hospital]. Flash said one run like that is worth a week of bullshit calls.

Even a failure, if the attendants perform well, can be considered a good run, though they might not adopt that view immediately. A crew who had a "code" in the ambulance, who did CPR on the way to the hospital, but who lost the patient would probably not want to talk about it right away.

Emergencies are more likely to be good runs than are nonemergencies. Runs that require efforts to control bleeding, the use of splints, antishock measures, and CPR allow the EMT to contribute actively to the patient's well-being. Runs that call for oxygen, suctioning, cold packs, or comfort are more routine but are still legitimate EMS work.

10:33 PM. We got a fire call to Golden State Drive. We were the only ones going in. [No rescue squad was available as first responder.] The patient was a very old woman sitting in a chair and smiling vaguely. Her elderly daughter said she had just got so she couldn't hold her cup of hot chocolate and didn't want to walk. Lyle told me to get the heart monitor. He cut her slip, attached the leads, and ran a tape. He made some reassuring comments and we put her on the cot, sitting up, and took her out to the rig. Lyle thought it was almost certainly a case of CHF [congestive heart failure] which would be accompanied by weak peripheral circulation, and possibly a related CVA [stroke] seen in the loss of motor skills indicated by the patient's plucking movements. We ran hot to County; the daughter rode up front. On the way Flash couldn't find a radial [wrist] pulse. Afterward Lyle said the heart waves were nearly flat. The patient's pulse was 28! It was amazing she was alive, incredible she was conscious, fantastic she was alert. He couldn't believe it. He saved a copy of the EKG tape for Jase.

Scheduled runs can be good, if they enable the EMT to learn something. The specialist from the Neonatal Critical Care Unit, who accompanies Liberty crews on baby calls, is happy to talk with them about the problems of newborns. And the scheduled transfer of a critical patient is often interesting because it is so complicated. On one occasion it was a Liberty EMT, crowded into the back with a physician, a nurse, and a respiratory therapist, who detected a leak around the patient's breathing tube.

Certain calls make an impression on the attendant without either involving him in life-saving efforts or generating much excitement. Something in the patient or in the event touches the attendant and causes him to turn reflective, as did The Doctor in the following example:

It was a typically slow Saturday afternoon. We were sprawled on the bunks in the Pit [the lavatory at the inactive Greyrock Community Hospital]. The Doctor told about a case they had the night before where a fourteen-year-old girl fell on the parallel bars and separated her shoulder. She was warming up for a meet, the really big one, and she slipped. She would have won the whole business; she was written up in all the papers. "Imagine how she felt! All that work and then she wasn't able to compete." The Doctor seemed to have a real feeling for her disappointment.

The attendant's sensitivity apparently depends upon his mood. Similar cases get a sympathetic response on one occasion and little notice on another. While the runs that produce these responses are not necessarily "good," the people involved do not consider them routine. But because of the you-had-to-be-there quality, the runs might well be dismissed as routine by those who only hear about them.

Nonemergency transfers, while they are not considered good runs by the crews, are not necessarily scorned. Though neither noteworthy nor demanding, they allow the attendants to provide a necessary service. A nonemergency transfer is satisfactory if it involves a good patient. A good patient is one who is cooperative and not demanding.[3] Of the types of practitioner-patient relations suggested by Szasz and Hollender, the EMT preference is closest to the "guidance-cooperation model," in which he directs and the patient complies by assuming correct body positions and answering questions.[4] The EMTs do not like patients who complain, who seem to exaggerate their discomfort, or who are emotionally out of control. Runs with these kinds of patients are stoically endured and quickly forgotten.

On a routine run with a good patient, the EMT is courteous and helpful, lifting and positioning the patient carefully, adjusting the cot and pillow. He complies with the patient's modesty by using a covering sheet and, if it is chilly, a blanket with a towel tucked around the head. It is not unusual for an attendant to act as the patient's advocate, asking a nurse to produce the patient's eyeglasses or assuring the patient that he has the false teeth, or the purse, or other special belongings. At times an attendant even serves as a counselor, as when Lyle sympathetically conferred with a woman who was dismayed at the thought of being returned to the nursing home and asked us not to take her. If the patient were unpleasant the quality of care could be adjusted downward enough to satisfy the attendant without provoking the patient further. The run would not then be thought of in a neutral way but would be classified as some kind of problem.

Shit Calls

A good run is celebrated by the EMTs, because so many of their calls are a waste of time. Barb's personal trip book, in which she listed her runs, showed that most were not medical emergencies. This condition is not peculiar to Metropolis. Surveys of city services elsewhere show that fewer than half the responses are for cases that really require an ambulance,[5] and that 15 to 30 percent of the runs of even paramedic units are nuisance calls.[6] Indeed the whole EMS system is being misused to some extent. Little more than half of the emergency room patients require attention within a few hours of their arrival, and only about 10 percent are true emergencies.[7] In the words of the company's medical advisor: "About 5 to 10 percent of the ER patients at County [Hospital] are emergency cases [true emergencies], another 10·percent are serious, and the other 80 percent are crap." Although the misuses of rigs and rooms are related, the benefits for the misusers are different. Both must deal with people who overestimate the seriousness of their conditions. Beyond that, ambulances seem to be summoned because they are convenient and cheap transportation (if insurance pays), because the attendants deliver a quick diagnosis, or even out of malicious mischief. Nuisance calls appear to be centered in low-income, high-density areas where people have learned to rely on public agencies, though some research suggests that in a particular service area the different social classes misuse emergency facilities at about the same rate.[8] This misuse evidently grows as people become more aware of the availability of EMS.

The occasions on which ambulances are summoned for nonemergency purposes are referred to variously as nonessential calls, abuse calls, nothing calls, nonemergency calls, and nuisance calls. The Liberty attendants refer to them as shit calls. Shit calls are by definition not good runs. The attendants do not think of the people who make these calls as patients.[9] They are nuisances who, mistakenly or cannily, are wasting the ambulance service's resources.

The EMTs have little patience for the ho-hum cases that could easily be handled by another means of transportation. These people may be acting out of genuine concern, but it is interpreted as excess caution by the attendants. They are called *walkers*, because they can walk to the ambulance and thereby prove they do not need it. (The English call such patients "sitting cases," because they sit up during the conveyance.)

3:15 PM. As soon as we cleared we got a scheduled call, lights and siren. It was described as a coronary thrombosis and I was worried that we were running hot because the patient was going sour. Flash thought Harold was sending us 10-17 because he had been sitting on the call and was trying to make up some time. The address was an up- stairs flat. Flash rang the bell and an elderly couple came down right away. The man, dressed in a bathrobe, looked pale and tired and wor- ried. The woman, who appeared to be more cheerful and generally healthier, was carrying an overnight bag. Flash and I took the man's arms and began helping him toward the ambulance, but he protested that his wife was the patient. She smiled and walked out to the rig. On the way to the hospital, she said she had wanted to wait until tomor- row but that her husband was worried about her.

The walker is a disappointment, because he reduces ambulance work to chauffeuring. The disappointment is heightened when the crew is antici- pating a good run, for example, at an accident. Accident victims are often walkers, but they are considered legitimate patients because of the trau- matic circumstances and the need for a thorough assessment. The EMTs admit the irony in dedicating themselves to health care and then being dis- satisfied at the lack of serious injuries.

More irritating to the crews are the *twenty-sevens,* a category derived from the company's code for bums and drunks. The twenty-sevens pos- sibly have a medical need, but they are interested in the ambulance pri- marily as a free means of conveyance. The crews recognize them by the combination of a lack of serious symptoms (though they often have chron- ic conditions) and a lack of convincing reasons for not taking alternative transportation. In effect they are walkers who want to ride but not pay. A taxi would demand a fare on the spot; with the ambulance they can make the trip, then ignore the bill or have it paid by Medicaid. In these cases it is often evident from the liquor and delicatessen food around that they do not suffer from a complete lack of money. A sizable portion of the twenty- sevens are *veterans* who want to go to the Veterans Administration Hospi- tal to continue treatments. They know the hospital, which has a contract with another private company (Towner), would not send an ambulance for them. So the family claims an emergency and calls the fire department, which routinely summons Liberty to make the transport if it is in their sec- tor. Unfortunately for Liberty, the VA usually refuses to pay for convey- ance other than by ambulances under contract to them. The crews often transport the caller to avoid the hassle of arguing, but they are disgusted at having to give in.

Some of the twenty-sevens have no money to pay for a taxi and are too fearful or unsteady to take a bus. They are classified as *bums.* The ambu- lance is usually summoned for them by proprietors (of flophouses or luncheonettes or the Rescue Mission) or by police who want to have the body removed from the premises. In effect, the police (or the firefighters) commit the private companies to hauling patients they might otherwise refuse. Unless the medical need is clear, which it rarely is, the crews resent what they consider this misuse by the police, because it implies that the ambulance is just a form of public transportation. The crews feel the bums could be carried by squad car or patrol wagon. They understand that the police do not want to be accused of mishandling a case, but they dislike the risk of running hot through city traffic without a medical reason. On the other side the police and firefighters on the scene suspect (no doubt correctly) that if the calls were not designated emergencies, the privates would be slow to respond. It is a further aggravation for the crews when emergency room personnel criticize them for bringing in bums with minor complaints for which the hospitals can do little.

Most of the twenty-sevens are *drunks.* Even the drunks with money are seldom paying customers. When they are sober they conclude that the ambulance ride was not necessary; their medical problems are rarely serious enough to be covered by insurance. The other services consider minor injuries from falling down, vomiting, even the confusion of the drunk, sufficient reason for calling an ambulance. The police give the hard cases a choice between going to jail or "voluntarily" signing themselves into the detoxification unit at the county hospital. One can never be sure what condition a drunk is in when he climbs into the rig.

11:45 PM. We got a 10-17 to the fountain at City-center. There were several police and firemen with a man down on his hands and knees complaining of chest pains. I thought we should get the cot, but Tanner figured he could walk. The man (45 yo w/m) was reluctant to go to the hospital; he specifically didn't want to go to VA. I put him on the squad bench and got a seat belt on him. His breath smelled powerfully of liquor. First he acted as though the ambulance were a paratroop plane. Then he told war stories about Korea. Then he leaned on my shoulder and cried. "Where has it all gone? How could such bright possibilities all vanish? What has happened?" It sounded like dialogue from a B movie. How much of it was on the level?

Hardly ever do the crews find the drunks amusing; usually they are messy and often difficult and belligerent.

Drunks not only waste their own resources, they involve other people in their havoc. Drunk-related devastation led John Riley to formulate his EMS Late Night Axiom: "If you respond to any accident after midnight and do not see a drunk, keep looking because someone is still missing."[10] Drunks are thought to be an important contributor to EMT burnout.

Because the same drunks turn up again and again, the crews have little hope of improving the situation. Too often the drunk will walk out of the hospital and be gone before the crew can finish the paperwork. The blame-the-patient tendency associated with burnout shows up in the abuse to which EMTs sometimes subject drunks. In an extreme case some frustrated EMTs gave a wino such a fierce ride it apparently precipitated a heart attack that killed him.[11] The Liberty attendants would occasionally give a drunk a rough ride (a code 10-71) but never a dangerous one. However, some of them harassed drunks by trying to confuse them.

EMT: *Well here we are in Baltimore finally.*
DRUNK: *What . . . how the fuck did I get to Baltimore? What are you talking about?*
EMT: *They didn't want you in Cleveland so we had to take you someplace.*
DRUNK: *Cleveland? Oh, no!*

EMT: *Whatever you do, don't let them catch you singing out at Detox.*
DRUNK: *Whatta you mean?*
EMT: *Seriously. It's a bad sign. The doctors don't like it. They took one guy's arm off because he was singing. He just woke up one morning and it was gone. He didn't know anything about it.*
DRUNK: *No shit!*

I heard it was only a few of the newer attendants who were heckling the patients. Jardine was disgusted at the idea; he said it "removed the dignity" from people. It was not only the privates that tormented the drunks.

Jase talked about their being called to transport a disoriented man who might have been drunk, too. Palermo [of the rescue squad] had bound his wrists with Kling since he was a bit violent. The Liberty crew got him in the rig and on the cot and calmed down a bit. Just before they closed the doors, Palermo ran up and shouted, "You're gonna die, fucker!" The patient went wild again. There were chuckles about Palermo. "That guy has balls. He'll do anything."

Whether the harassment is interpreted as a consequence of sadism or of simple frustration, it indicates that some of the attendants have ceased to think of the drunks as patients.

Walkers and twenty-sevens, while they do not require an ambulance, are at least incapacitated to some extent. Many of the shit calls are people whom the crews suspect have no medical problem at all. It is hard to substantiate these suspicions because the patients use a range of symptoms that cannot be measured. Even though the vital signs show no abnormality, the attendants cannot dismiss the other symptoms. The patients claim weakness, dizziness, nerves acting up, shortness of breath, persistent pain, and nausea. They demonstrate their discomfort by breathing rapidly, moaning, coughing, the dry heaves (gagging without vomiting), crying hysterically, and even fainting. Sometimes a patient will ask "Where am I?" in a surprised voice so unconvincing it is all the EMTs can do to keep from laughing out loud. The crews' suspicions are strengthened when they see the emergency room staff's reactions to these patients—much frowning, rolling of eyes, looking disgusted, shaking of heads, and barely civil greetings. To add to the difficulty, there are patients with genuine medical problems, such as asthma and emphysema, that cannot be adequately treated by the emergency services. These patients do not falsify their symptoms, but they are as much a bother as those who do.

The crews form a clear impression about the lack of medical need of those patients who misuse the service again and again. The crews call them *regulars*.

3:54 PM. We got a fire call, no rescue squad going in. A bearded man in T-shirt and bermudas greeted Flash like an old friend and led us up some outside stairs to the first floor. The patient (22 yo w/f) complained of stomach pains, nausea, vomiting, and diarrhea. She stressed that she had eaten some potato salad last night. The man insisted on an ambulance. They had a Title 19 card [Medicaid]. As we walked her out to the rig she shouted, "Get those people away from here! I don't want them looking at me!" Flash said in a quiet voice, "There's not much we can do about that." At the hospital the ED nurse seemed to recognize the patient. "You're also diabetic, aren't you?" Outside Flash told me the patient was a regular and this was a bullshit call. I'm so new I can't recognize them, and even if I could, there's no way to avoid treating them if they demand it.

The fire department dispatchers learn to know the regulars and call for a private ambulance without sending a rescue squad. The attendants talk about the regulars with a mixture of contempt (because they are a bother) and fascination (because they have the audacity to continue their games). They talk about the large girl who is paralyzed from the waist down and who can roll her eyes back and simulate respiratory arrest, and the bearded crazy who calls at three in the morning and when the ambulance arrives says he does not want to be transported. The attendants shake their heads and cluck over them as they might over embarrassing relatives. "We took Chester Weber to Zion today. I think he just might die on us. Chet is beginning to look pretty funky. They say he's had a lot of urinary tract infections."

The regulars evidently play at being sick not because of the medical treatment itself (which is apparently ineffective) but because of secondary gains in the treatment process. If they feel neglected and lonely, they can have the attention of the medical personnel; if they are bored, they can escape their daily routine; if they are troubled by other problems, the medical procedures can be distracting and reassuring; if they feel powerless, they can use their disability to manipulate others. These people create adventures out of their experiences by fabricating details. A twenty-five-year-old woman who regularly calls for help for a variety of elusive symptoms tells the attendants about the fireman who saved her life by doing CPR on her. She even names him, though the rescue squads can never verify that such a person exists.

Eventually the hospital personnel tell the ambulance companies not to bring specific regulars back. Their primary reason is that the hospitals cannot help them. A second reason is that the patients cannot pay for the services. Thus, those who were once received as paying patients become nonpaying nuisances. It is more difficult for the company to disengage itself from regulars. Some regulars contact the fire department and Liberty must respond to these emergency calls; some contact the company directly. Haroid was furious when he learned Noah Blue (a regular) had a Liberty stick-on phone label. When he tried to find out where he had gotten it, Jardine suggested it might have been from a competitor. Flash thought we should give him a stick-on from another company.

Similar to the regulars are what might be called *repeaters,* though the Liberty crews do not use this term. The repeaters make multiple uses of the ambulances for doubtful cause, but instead of developing a long-term pattern they bunch their calls.

10:25 AM. A fire call. Jase and Sonya were next up but Flash said we'd take it. We ran hot to N. Burgess with Vic riding as third man. The patient (37 yo b/f) was lying on the sofa in the living room. She complained of pains on the left side of her head, neck, shoulder, and side when she stood up. She was able to walk to the ambulance; her husband rode in front. I got the general information while Vic took her vitals, which were normal. The nurse at Mercy recognized the husband. She told me, "But they were just in here yesterday! For the husband! What are we going to do with them? (Look of exasperation.) I guess it's not you guys' fault." She said there was no medical reason for them to be there.

8:50 PM. Fire call for N. Burgess, where we had been this morning. Flash and Dixie took it because Flash had been there before. He told us the problem was supposed to be pregnancy this time. "Another bullshit call," he said as they left.

During one three-week period Liberty was called to the same place at least three times (and probably more since different crews were involved) for different problems, none medically serious. Strangely, the callers gave the wrong house number every time; they always asked for an ambulance for 104, which did not exist; the patient was always at 140. The repeaters act as though they have discovered a new game and are trying out its possibilities before they tire of it.

The final category of shit calls is that of the *fakers*. These are people who, for whatever reason, get themselves involved in an ambulance call and then put on a show to justify it. Since they have not developed a record of abuse like the regulars and repeaters, the crews cannot be sure about them. One behavior that arouses suspicion is an emotional display—loud groaning or hysterical crying—out of all proportion to the known injury. The crews' biases also color their assessment of the patients; if they like the patient, they assume a real injury, if not they suspect faking. The crews' classifications of patients are summarized in Figure 6-1.

The crews realize that many unnecessary runs are due to the over-reaction of concerned families and friends who panic when confronted by

Figure 6-1

AMBULANCE ATTENDANTS' CLASSIFICATION OF PATIENTS

		Able to Pay	*Not Able to Pay*
Requires Ambulance		Good Run	Good Run

Shit Calls

		Walker	(Twenty-seven) Bum Drunk
Does Not Require Ambulance	*Possible Medical Need*	Walker	(Twenty-seven) Bum Drunk
	Doubtful Medical Need	Regular	Repeater Faker

an unexpected medical problem. Some face questions without answers: should a known epileptic be taken to a hospital after a seizure? Public standards for judging emergencies are particularly shaky in Metropolis, where until recently the police transported all emergency calls free with no questions asked. During the first six months of the new EMS system, the privates conveyed only half the number of patients the police had transported for a comparable period the year before. The difference was supposedly due to the new fees for ambulance rides and to screening by the crews. The unnecessary runs of a better-safe-than-sorry sort reinforce the crews' cynicism about the public's knowledge of medical care generally and of ambulance services in particular. However, it is the calculated abuse calls, where they feel someone is trying to make fools of them, that make them angry.

The cynicism and anger of the attendants emerge in their treatment of the patients. When they think a patient is faking, they will challenge him. They will take a set of vitals and use the results to talk him out of going to the hospital. If he claims dizziness or appears to faint, they will use ammonia inhalants or painful pinches to return him to normal. If the patient claims a stomach or abdominal disorder or even a mild drug problem, they will predict that the hospital will require having his stomach pumped or an enema. If the patient persists in demanding transportation, the attendants will usually comply but will try to make the ride unrewarding. Inverting the common decision rule, they will assume a best-case rather than a worst-case scenario by minimizing the importance of the problem and taking shortcuts. They will have the patient walk to the ambulance rather than use the wheeled cot; they will have the patient sit on the squad bench rather than lie down; they will tell the patient they have no oxygen on board or that the air conditioner will be sufficient; they will take the patient to a hospital of their convenience rather than his. If possible, they will give the patient a rough ride, and the tech in back will endure the discomfort out of spite.

On rare occasions, usually as a result of fatigue, one of the attendants will "flood out" and completely reject the medical definition of the situation.[12] He will deny that a genuine problem exists, blame the patient for whatever problem is claimed, and refuse to give any help. He might even threaten the patient.

7:55 AM. Louie called to say he would be late. The sound of the new crews coming in woke Flash. He telephoned Harold to tell him he blew up at a patient last night. As the story came out, a friend claimed the patient was shell-shocked. Flash lost control and got furious, though he doesn't know exactly what set him off. Jardine intervened but Flash refused to be in the same rig with the patient; he wouldn't even drive

and let Jardine tech. Finally Jardine radioed for another ambulance.
The Doctor, who was on the backup rig, said the patient was having
flashbacks from his Vietnam experiences. He would yell, "In-coming!
In-coming!" and fall to the ground shrieking and holding on with
everything he had. He had visions of a buddy torn to shreds. The Doc-
tor said the guy was no longer in Metropolis, he was back in the war. [13]
The Doctor came on like a medic [which he actually had been, though
not in Vietnam], and handled the patient that way.

In these situations the other attendant acts as mediator and might be able
to use seniority to control the event. If that is not possible, the breakdown
of the run becomes known to others through the call for assistance. Usually
the EMT who floods out is shaken by the experience and contrite, but
those who do not have an otherwise strong record with the company are
not likely to survive such a serious breach of regulations.

Problems of Control

Unlike emergency departments in hospitals, the ambulances cannot screen
out nuisance calls before initiating service. It is not until they are on the
scene that they can determine that the "man down" is really a drunk sound
asleep. Since ambulances are relatively expensive to operate and hence
few in number, each nuisance call reduces the number of cars available to
handle genuine emergencies. Abuse calls are therefore more than a bother
for the crews; they are a danger to the community, because they diminish
the effectiveness of the EMS system.

Logically, the first line of defense by EMS systems would be *education of*
the public about the nature and limits of ambulance service and about how
to recognize emergencies. Unfortunately it is nearly impossible to train a
whole city population, for example, to distinguish serious from not so serious medical problems. Moreover, the determined abusers would not be
deterred. Where they have been tried, public education programs have increased the visibility of the EMS system, and as the case load subsequently
increased so did the abuse calls.[14] Metropolis has never had a public information program on EMS, even though some of the private companies
have asked for it.

The second line of defense against system abuse is the *dispatcher*. Experienced dispatchers are able to identify the calls that are obviously unnecessary or nuisances and handle them without sending a car. Dispatcher
training, together with the use of uniform procedures and formal protocols, car increase the value of this kind of screening.[15] But screening by
telephone has serious limitations. Determined abusers learn to describe the
right symptoms (for example, pain in the chest and left shoulder, which

suggests a heart attack) to insure that an ambulance will be sent. The dispatcher has to give the benefit of the doubt to the caller, for if he makes a mistake and treats a true emergency as a nuisance call, he risks his job, his reputation, and even prosecution.[16] The cost of such mistakes to the dispatcher and to his organization is so high that the tendency is to roll first and ask questions later. Liberty, because it receives its emergency calls from the fire department dispatcher, is not able to do its own screening.

The third line of defense against abuse is screening by the *crew* on the scene. While they have a better basis for estimating the seriousness of the case than does the dispatcher, even they cannot be certain. Apparently benign conditions may be evidence of more severe problems—a nose bleed of hypertension, for example, or scalp laceration of concussion —and some patients minimize their discomfort, like the mangled motorcyclist in the well-worn story, who regained consciousness momentarily and asked only if his bike was OK. The fact that attendants sometimes disagree about the seriousness of the complaint, or sometimes concentrate on different symptoms, increases the difficulty of screening. The necessity of screening puts the EMT into something of an adversary relationship with the patient, a complication that is avoided if all calls are transported without question. This adversary stance is not predominant, however; attendants often encourage reluctant patients to go to the hospital and transport even doubtful cases if the patient is infirm, without family support, hindered by bad weather, or lacking other means of transportation.

The strongest pressure on the crews in the field is to convey the patient. The fact that they are on the scene means they have already invested something in the run, and it will cost little more to complete it. The family and bystanders want to see action. And, like the dispatchers, the crews must consider the consequences of making a mistake. One of the Metropolis privates (not Liberty) was attacked by the newspapers for not conveying a man who was later found to have acute meningitis, even though apparently he had not consented to go to a hospital.[17] In addition, the EMTs working for private companies feel an obligation to make the run profitable. Whether the patient can pay, which is never certain until the money is in the bank, is another criterion that becomes part of the screening, if only informally. The Liberty crews acknowledge it with mild cynicism: "Should we transport if the patient has $75 [the rate at the time] but no medical need?" Some of them transport anyone who insists using the rationale that "in this business the company has to give something away once in a while." Once it is decided that they will transport, the tech will report the patient's condition in terms most likely to convince insurers. He will play up signs and symptoms possibly related to critical conditions, such as shock, heart attack, serious blood loss, or brain damage, and will deemphasize chronic conditions or minor symptoms. In doing so, the tech is trying to mislead the insurance claims adjuster in the same way the nuisance caller is trying to mislead the dispatcher.

A fourth line of defense is the *financial charge* for the run. The introduction of a fee for ambulance services has helped reduce the total number of runs in Metropolis. However, many of the abusers are covered by Medicare, Medicaid, or other insurance, and thus are little affected by the cost. The state legislature once tried to establish a mandatory fee to be charged by hospital emergency departments in order to discourage misuse, but it was not able to carry out the plan.

A fifth defense, in which local ordinances set *fines* and *prison terms* for people convicted of misusing ambulance services, shows promise but has not yet been thoroughly tested. Until effective controls are found, ambulance workers will continue to bear the tiresome burden of shit calls.

The Dead and the Dying

The crews do not like to handle dead bodies. Not only do the bodies not require medical services, they threaten unpleasant surprises because of decomposition. Consequently, runs that involve the dead are almost inevitably shit calls. There are exceptions, of course, and the degree of distaste varies with the attendant's personal background, the scene, and the nature of the attendant's participation. The Doctor, for example, because of a very bad experience in childhood, has a personal reason for loathing any contact with a corpse, while other attendants feel less repugnance. Whatever their personal attitudes, however, the crews find the emotional demonstrations of the survivors a burden; to load and run is less trying than to prepare a body for transport in the presence of weeping relatives. Finally, if the crew helps to fight the death, the run is not a shit call. As crew members took the body of a man off the factory floor, where they had worked on him for an hour with the paramedics, one of the workers said, "Thanks for doing what you could, fellas." That was not a thoroughly good run, but neither was it a thoroughly bad one.

The dead present the crews not only with physical and emotional messes, but also with definitional problems. For the EMTs the line between the dead and the dying is ambiguous. This is sometimes true in a clinical sense when the physical assessment is unclear; it is nearly always true in a legal sense. The ambiguity follows from the law that only certain persons (usually a physician or coroner) are authorized to pronounce someone dead or to sign the death certificate. In a technical sense even the most unmistakably dead are legally alive until they have been officially "pronounced." Presumably this means that in such a case an EMT's decision not to begin CPR could be legally challenged, since he is obligated to prevent further deterioration in a patient's condition until someone else takes over responsibility.[18] The decision not to act, however reasonable a judgment, may be a tacit (and unauthorized) pronouncement of death. The ambiguity puts the crews in an awkward situation on the scene if they consider a patient dead but cannot use that description with the family. They are forced to use evasions ("I'm sorry but there's nothing we can do for him."). Informally the EMTs use the term "DOE"—dead on entry—to refer to a corpse, but on the EMT report they formally present the case as a "pulseless nonbreather" or as a "possible DOE."

When a patient has just died, the EMT's decisions are even more difficult. Under most conditions a patient who has been in cardiac or respiratory arrest for less than six minutes will be considered revivable and, in effect, dying rather than dead.[19] The attendants rarely know exactly how long a patient has been a pulseless nonbreather, however, and must therefore make a judgment about whether to initiate CPR. In Metropolis, where the rescue squads are the first responders and paramedics are summoned in life-threatening cases, the private EMTs are not often forced to make such decisions. From their stories and conversations though, the Liberty attendants seem to use the same criteria Sudnow found important in emergency rooms—they would be more hesitant to initiate resuscitation on the very old and on those of apparently low socioeconomic circumstances (bums) or of questionable moral character (drunks, drug abusers).[20] These criteria are reinforced when the crews hear ED physicians comment on cases in which CPR was not successful: "He was young and healthy. We shouldn't have lost him." The only criterion that is part of the formal training program teaches that CPR is not indicated for "a patient who is known to be in the terminal stages of an incurable illness."[21] One course instructor put it in a more folksy way: "If they are very old and sick, let them go. You won't do anyone a favor by trying to hold on to them." Clearly it would be absurd to require EMTs to use CPR in all cases where the body has not been formally pronounced dead. Yet anything short of that forces the EMT to use his discretion and raises ethical questions about how one should determine whether to attempt to revive a patient. In emergencies there is no time for consultation or for a committee decision.

There is one situation in which the attendants can always be expected to initiate CPR—when the patient "codes" (becomes a pulseless nonbreather) in the back of the ambulance. Here the EMT has formal responsibility and knows exactly when the patient arrested. But even under these conditions, there is opportunity for the play of individual judgment.

Louie said Jardine had let a patient die in the back of the ambulance. It was a terminal cancer patient, a man who was so much like a skeleton he was painful to look at. He was evidently suffering a lot as well.

They were on the way to St. Christopher's with the man's wife in front. She looked pretty wrung out, too. Louie was driving and noticed that Jardine had switched to the [dim] blue lights in back. Louie asked if everything was alright and got a short affirmative. When they got to St. Chris Jardine told Louie to walk the wife into the admitting area first and then come back to help with the cot. At that point Louie knew that something was wrong. When he got back to the rig, Jardine told him the patient was dead. They took him into the ED where the staff was a bit startled by Jardine's report, but they didn't try to revive the patient either. The ED physician told Jardine privately that he had done the right thing, that there was no point in trying to keep the man alive. Jardine's hesitance to resuscitate was not based on any aversion; he had done CPR a lot of other times. It was a deliberate decision. The question is whether he had the right to decide.

Most attendants probably would not have the inclination or the courage to do what Jardine did. Theirs would be an automatic response to perform CPR until they arrived at the hospital. In some cases Jardine's action would be seen as a service to everyone; in others it might be seen as a dereliction of duty.[22]

This discussion points up a problem of contemporary society. Since the improvement of emergency medical services, it has become more difficult for people to die. Once the family decides to call in the medical care system, the patient is handed from one service to another, with each doing its best to stave off death. For example, a nursing home will summon an ambulance rather than allow a patient to die on the premises. The ambulance crew will keep the patient alive by using basic life support. The emergency room staff will attempt to revive the patient. And the hospital will then use support systems to lengthen the patient's survival. But where in all this is the recognition that death is inevitable and even appropriate? Who shall decide that it is the right time for death? Informally the decisions are made when medical personnel do less than the maximum to sustain certain patients or when "reasonable" efforts (which can vary from ten minutes of CPR for one patient to more than an hour for others) seem to be ineffective. As we have seen, in some circumstances even EMTs make these decisions.

Tunas

Ambulance workers will tell you that all patients are heavy, but some are heavier than others. The Liberty attendants call outstandingly hefty patients "tunas."

5:50 PM. We got a call to go to South Hatcher to back up Jase and The Doctor. Flash said those two are among the strongest in the company. If they need help it must be a real tuna. The patient was on the second floor (naturally) of a house with a long porch stair (no railing) and a narrow, steep inside stair with a ceiling so low a normal person had to stoop. The Doctor said later this was the first time he ever had to call for a backup. Flash said this was the biggest person he ever had to move. The patient (45 yo Amerindian or Polynesian/m) had supposedly been sitting in an easy chair for two days unable to move. He reported that he had cirrhosis of the liver and other organic difficulties, and he had a sore with edema on his right leg involving the knee. Flash figured the patient's ankles were about the size of his [Flash's] thighs. Later estimates of the patient's weight ranged from 350 to 600 pounds. We used the folding stretcher with the wheels and legs down. The patient was reluctant to give up his can of beer to be moved! The Doctor put it on a side table where the wife later knocked it over. Getting him out of the chair into which he was well sunk was tough. I had his extremely painful right leg to both lift and guide. It was hot up there, and while we were shifting him a fan kept blowing the Chux off the stretcher. The wife, who was rather detached and vaguely giggly throughout the proceedings, turned it off. We were all covered with sweat when we got done. Finally we got him onto the stretcher and strapped down. Just as we are ready to move him downstairs he asks for his cough drops. Cough drops! The Doctor exclaims, "Man, the question is whether you're going to get down those stairs alive. Don't worry about cough drops." "Alive?" the man asks, his attention at last having focused on the problem at hand. "Have you looked at your stairs lately?", The Doctor replies. The Doctor figured those cough drops might be the straw that would break all our backs. The Doctor and Flash went down first, backwards, with the foot of the stretcher. Jase and I were at the head, pulling back. Jase was worried that I would get knocked off the railingless porch with him and the patient landing on top of me. We got him down onto the gurney, folded the stretcher wheels and braces under, and put it all in the rig. Everyone was panting. Flash and I cleared at 6:10.

The tunas represent a sizable category in which patients are remembered primarily as problems. Although they may have genuine medical needs, these patients present such notable nonmedical difficulties as sheer *weight*.[23] The crews are equally impressed by having to maneuver in awkward settings, calm emotional cases, and cope with people who are reluctant to go to the hospital.

The inconvenience of *setting* may be due to narrow and turning stairs, cold and wet and cramped quarters (for example, a sewer manhole and tunnel), hindrance in gaining access to the patient (perhaps trapped in a crushed automobile), or danger (such as a walkway on the verge of collapsing). Lack of light is always an impediment, and filth is always a bother. One of the memorable cases at Liberty was a recluse who lived in a junk-filled apartment with an assortment of dogs and cats and no electricity. The rescue squad summoned to her dark, reeking flat eagerly handed the job over to the Liberty attendants, who had to wade through urine-soaked newspapers, around tottering piles of cartons, and past starving animals to locate and lift the raving woman out of a back corner. Although the attendants used gloves and paper sheets, they were not able to protect themselves from the muck and the stench, which followed them the rest of the day. The case was a benchmark for miserable conditions.

Other patients are problems because of their *attitudes*. Some are complainers and others are whiners. The complainers bewail the cause of their difficulty, the person they think is to blame, and the inadequate service of everyone connected with medical care. One woman, who had cut her scalp when the bus stopped suddenly, complained to her husband about his "idiotic" decision to leave the car, about the bloodstain on her new suit, about the ruin of her hairdo, and about the bumpy ambulance ride. The crew pitied the unfortunate ED aide who would have to shave the woman's head. The whiners seem to be exploiting a legitimate medical need in order to satisfy an urge to be dependent. They regress to childlike behavior, crying and calling for help. A woman who had been hit over the head with a flowerpot whimpered. "I want to die! Just let me die!" A man responsible for an automobile accident that injured a little girl (but not seriously) raved about how he deserved to die and refused any treatment from the EMTs, though he allowed them to take him to a hospital. Another woman, picked up in front of a bar with fingers that appeared to have been broken by having a door slammed on them, called repeatedly to her surly companion in the front of the rig, "Bobby, help me! My fingers are getting numb! Bobby!" Demonstrative people sound much like fakers to the attendants and as a result may be taken less seriously at times than their conditions warrant.

The crews attempt to get these disturbed patients under control by showing them that something is being done for them. Often the EMT has little beyond a cold pack that can directly affect the patient's condition. But sometimes the appearance of treatment alone is enough, as when a weeping child is calmed by having his cut covered with a Band-aid. The crews use a variety of techniques as placebos to comfort distraught patients.[24] Providing pillows and loosening already loose seat belts, putting nasal cannulas in place without activating the oxygen supply, telling the patient to take slow, deep breaths, and even attaching the leads for the heart monitor can help in getting the patient under control.

Patients who have a probable medical need but who are *reluctant* to go to the hospital are a more serious problem. They may be depressed, undergoing drug reactions, disoriented, or manifestly suicidal. The attendants usually support bystanders in trying to coax the patient to be checked out by a physician, but if he is not willing, there is little anyone can do about it. Occasionally the police will pressure a drunk into going to the hospital ("Which will it be, jail or the detoxification center?"), but there is no guarantee he will stay around for treatment. In certain circumstances—attempted suicide or a psychotic episode, for example—the police may take a patient into custody and have him transferred to a hospital under their auspices.

Patient Consent

The law emphasizes the patient's right to refuse treatment.[25] Therefore the EMT must be careful not to take any action without the consent of the patient or someone legally responsible for him. In the case of conscious adults, the consent should be express and voluntary. When upset family members called a Liberty ambulance for a woman whose erratic drinking and eating habits had resulted in a deteriorating of her behavior and in her wasting away to 80 pounds, the crew did not doubt that she needed help. But when they were told she would refuse to go to the hospital with them, they did not even leave the ambulance. They felt they could only advise the family to contact a lawyer or the Legal Aid Society to help have her treated under involuntary consent established by the process of law. As the company attendants often expressed it, to transport a patient like that against her will would be kidnapping. A notice on the Station 2 bulletin board made the position explicit: "Do not transport prisoners or incapacitated persons without incapacitation papers from the M.P.D. [Metropolis Police Department]. Otherwise it's kidnapping!" The other side of the coin is the risk of turning down a needy patient. In the case of acute meningitis mentioned above (and in note 17), the man refused to let the EMTs examine him, and they interpreted his behavior to mean that he did not want to go with them. The man's mother, who was on the scene, maintained that he did not know what he was doing. But it is difficult, according to a lawyer-paramedic, for an ambulance crew to determine when a reluctant patient should be understood as giving implied consent.[26]

Tearaway Ties

In the same way that some patients are thought of as nuisances and others as problems, a few patients are thought of as dangers. When the company first undertook EMS work, the uniform included a dress shirt and black necktie under the smock. Because a disturbed patient might grab the tie and use it in an attack, the attendants were instructed to wear clip-on ties that would tear away if pulled. Liberty eventually abandoned the shirt and tie for daily work, but the tearaway remains a symbol of the danger patients can represent for the attendants.

Ambulance workers face nonspecific threats constantly. There is the remote but real possibility of contracting a disease or infection from a patient's scratch or from airborne organisms. Excited pets, particularly dogs, are a hazard. Private settings where there has been violence—sexual assault, family beatings, fights—promote a sense of peril insofar as the assailant might return. Even settings not connected with specific incidents arouse the attendants' anxiety. Dark alleys, Gino's Bar with its rough crowd, the black ghetto at night, "Little Puerto Rico," where a crew was caught in a summer riot—all set off warning signals in the minds of the Liberty crews.

The attendants also encounter particular individuals or situations that are threatening. One of the most frequent is the belligerent drunk who challenges them. The emotionally unstable, called "looney-toons" by many of the crews, are sometimes threatening. A greater threat comes from people who are hostile but neither unsteady nor disoriented. For example, a Chicago paramedic suffered severe and permanent injury when an enraged husband of a patient threw him against the curb.[27] The worst are the hostiles with weapons. One of the policeman's most hated calls is "barricaded subject with gun," and occasionally the attendants run into just such a situation. One sunny afternoon Jase and his partner were met on the sidewalk by a caller who said her husband was disturbed and breaking things inside the house. They headed inside until she mentioned that he had a gun with him. They backed the ambulance out of range and called in a 10-53 (request for police). Within twenty minutes the quiet street was swarming with plainclothesmen. Flash claimed to have been pinned down by gunfire that destroyed a beacon on the ambulance. Jardine and his partner once had to back down a set of stairs, sweating and on the edge of panic, while they watched the barrel of a shotgun wavering in their faces.

Dealing with Danger

The most prevalent technique of self-protection is *prudence*. The crews take a cautious approach to other threatening situations just as they practice defensive driving when they are running hot. They use stereotypes in sizing up scenes and people to determine whether they need to stay close together, for example, or whether they should call for help.[28] They learn such precautions as standing to the side of a doorway when they knock. (Jilly told people that a partner of hers was killed by a shotgun blast through a door.) They are even wary of retaliation from disgruntled patients. Some attendants refuse to wear nameplates through which they could be traced, and Pete got an unlisted phone number to escape harassing calls. The overall strategy is to anticipate danger and avoid it, or at least limit its consequences.

The attendants supposedly prepare for danger, too, by arming themselves. Some of them have *devices or tactics* that could be used to subdue troublemakers.[29] There was the heavy flashlight Jardine carried and the wrist-lock holds and martial arts moves tried out in quarters. Since no one reported using these techniques, their primary contribution may have been to boost the confidence of the EMTs. What the attendants actually do in the face of danger is less dramatic. They usually rely on *persuasion*, talking quietly to get the patient to calm down and cooperate, as Jase did in dealing with the big "psycho" who threatened to throw him out of the rig. On that occasion Jase, among other things, opened the oxygen supply valve and convinced the patient the ambulance would blow up if the patient tried to light a cigarette. The attendants also use the gurney straps and the seat belts as *restraints* to keep the patients under control. On rare occasions they might use bandages or slings to limit a patient's movements. None of the Liberty attendants carry handcuffs, though employees of other private companies sometimes do.

It is perfectly acceptable to call for *police protection* when weapons or other specific dangers are involved. Such calls can in fact become routine for particular settings. The Liberty crews will not enter Gino's Bar unless the police are on the scene. However, such precautions must be carefully coordinated and will add to the time required for a run. In Chicago a paramedic team reluctant to enter a public-housing complex waited for 29 minutes for a police squad to rendezvous with them; by then the patient was dead. A week later a similar event occurred when a man allegedly told a paramedic crew entering the building for a heart attack case that if his "mother died, the crew would not leave the building alive." The paramedics retreated, and while they waited for an escort, the woman died.[30]

The hostility, threats, and injuries received by EMS personnel in certain cities (though not noticeably in Metropolis) seem to have several sources: racism—the suspect sectors are usually minority areas and the attendants are usually white; poverty—the poor blame the Establishment for their plight and the ambulance workers represent the Establishment; divergent definitions of the situation—the attendants associate the sectors with nuisance calls and the residents resent the attendants' refusals to transport. Added to this discord is the aggravation for both parties of the slower responses that are almost inevitable when two or more services collaborate.

The inconsistency of allowing units to enter these sectors unescorted if they are willing does not help much; it sets the scene for failed expectations. Perhaps it would be more efficient to arm the EMTs, as is already done in some squads under the auspices of law enforcement agencies. However, this suggestion would no doubt create serious problems of conscience for many of the EMTs.

The Effects of Social Status

Attendants categorize runs according to medical need or special problems, but they also notice the social status of their patients. A few universally recognized characteristics—age, gender, socioeconomic class, and ethnic background—help to determine how the patient is treated. Moreover, the attendant's own status affects his perceptions and responses. Social status influences both the attendant's style of relating to the patient and his estimate of the patient's condition. The consistency of the behavior of the Liberty personnel in this regard is partly due to the fact that most of them are young males from middle-class, white families.

Status is inevitably assessed in terms of age and gender. With regard to *age,* each patient is quickly classified as child, young adult, adult, or old person, and the attendant's behavior is guided by that classification. Because few of the attendants have their own, they handle children more by inclination than by skill; they are genuinely concerned but somewhat awkward. The interaction is complicated by the children's families, who often require more comfort than the children themselves. Further, since children are relatively easy to move, it is rarely essential to have an ambulance take them to a hospital. Again it is the families who, because of panic (or because of a crafty working-the-system), unnecessarily summon the ambulance and put the child and the attendants in an awkward position. The attendants almost always transport children; only in the most blatant instances of misuse do they refuse them.

The attendants are especially aware of young adults because they are age-mates and because they rarely are ambulance patients (except for certain kinds of vehicle accidents). Interaction with young adults is likely to be more lively and more prolonged than with other patients, and to include more joking and even some flirting. Young adults usually do not fabricate symptoms, and in life-threatening cases the crews seem to feel a special urgency to help them, perhaps because it seems so inappropriate that they should die. Since the attendant can realistically feel he is equal or superior in status to young adults and children, the appropriate forms of interaction are fairly clear.

With other adults, both the proper form of interaction and the medical need are ambiguous. How, for example, should an attendant address a patient who is older than he: formally, to seem polite, or informally, to seem friendly?[31] Because terms of address indicate relative status,[32] the attendants can and do use them to establish the subordinate position of the patient. They often use the first name of the patient in the familiar manner they would with children; the patient cannot even reciprocate because he does not know the attendant's name. The crews also carry a suspicious attitude about medical need into their relations with this age group, because it provides most of their nuisance calls.

The attendants call nearly all elderly patients by their first names.[33] Jilly claims the patients want it that way, that it makes them feel more trusting and comfortable. Barb says she's had occupational therapy patients who assumed she was being unfriendly because she called them "Mister." The other side of this assumption is seen in a nursing home resident telling the nurse who called her "Tillie" that her name is Matilda. What seems to one person to be friendly, may seem to another to be a theft of dignity. The attendants are less certain about how to evaluate the elderly medically. Some will record an upset patient as "confused," while others consider an incoherent person to be "normal."[34] Perhaps because many of the elderly patients do not make specific responses (sometimes due to hearing loss or confusion), the attendants are inclined to treat them more casually than they would others, for instance, making remarks about them in their presence. At the same time, the crews never express repugnance for the elderly, unlike the intern who said he could never bring himself to do resuscitation by putting his mouth to "an old lady's like that."[35]

Neither men nor women get preferential treatment, but *gender* is important in certain circumstances. There are no particular problems when attendants and patients are of the same gender, nor is there much difficulty when attendants must deal with members of the opposite sex who are much younger or much older than they. The men will routinely cut an elderly woman's slip to attach heart monitor leads, and the women will routinely check under an elderly man's sheets to see if there is a Foley catheter in place. However, patients who are nearly the same age can cause the EMTs to become self-conscious and hesitant. Once when a Liberty crew and a rescue squad were treating a young woman who had severely scalded herself, five men avoided any move to deal with the burns on her thighs and legs until the oldest of them opened her trousers and pulled them down. Thus can problems in interaction create problems in care. In urgent cases, such as emergency childbirth, the fact that the attendants might be male is not a serious impediment. At other times there are advantages to having attendant and patient be of the same gender; Barb is much more adept than the men at dealing with menstrual problems.

It may be true that the upper classes benefit less from emergency medical services because they are inclined to ignore ambulance crews in favor of their family physicians and thus sacrifice valuable time and skills. Among the rest of the public who do call on them, however, the EMTs distinguish several *socioeconomic classes*. In Liberty's sector, which encompasses a variety of neighborhoods, from slums to riverside mansions, the crews recognize bums, freaks, workers, respectable people, and notables. These distinctions are based on the patient's appearance and on his neighborhood. The crews are slightly more formal with people who are apparently of higher economic standing—when they took a man out of one of Metropolis's finest restaurants, they called him "Sir." The patients beneath the upper crust are treated more familiarly and some of them considerably less civilly. Moreover, insofar as context affects diagnosis,[36] estimated class has an effect on patient care. The crews divide the city into areas associated with different kinds of patients—"the Marina" (wealthy), "Little Africa" (poor blacks), "Looneyland" (drug overdoses, psychos, attempted suicides), "the low-rent district" (bums, drunks), "the tracts" (middle classes), "the industrial valley" (workers), "the towers" (elderly).[37] A crew going into one of these areas anticipates that the patient will fit a stereotype, and he will be treated accordingly unless there is clear reason to do otherwise. A complaint of stomach cramps in Looneyland may be dismissed as chronic imagination more quickly than in a different setting. At the least, alternative means of transportation would be suggested more quickly.

Many of the neighborhood stereotypes are based on the predominant *ethnic background* of the residents. The most obvious ethnic characteristics are language and color. None of the Liberty attendants know a foreign language, though a minority of their runs involve Spanish-speaking patients. The language barrier makes communication nearly impossible and disrupts patient care. The company puts Spanish phrase books in each trauma box, but when the attendants need them they have difficulty finding them, and when they find them they have difficulty using them. The effects of color, that is, racial prejudice, are less readily determined. Most of the time there is no evidence in the attendants' behavior of discourtesy or discrimination based on race. But now and then in quarters racism surfaces in an outpouring of jokes and slurs against blacks, expressed in slang terms ("jigaboos," "porch monkeys"), in exaggerated expressions ("Dis hear is a ee-mergency."), and in degrading suggestions ("Once you try black, you'll never go back."). The owners appear to share these attitudes, for example, Harold described twenty-sevens as "drunks, bums, niggers, whatever you want to call them." Some attendants express equally strong feelings in milder terms: "I guess there are reasons why they need all those fancy leather coats and still live like that [in squalor]." The occasions for such comments are brief, infrequent, and limited to only about half of the crews, but they indicate at least a lack of sympathy that could be expected to affect patient care. Again, as in the case of class, modifications of practice in response to ethnic status seem to be limited to the evaluation of questionable cases and perhaps to the style of interaction. However, assuming a patient's complaint to be minor because of his ethnic background—for example, having her walk to the rig in spite of a pain in the hip—could lead to complications in some instances.

The attendant's behavior is affected by his estimate of the patient's social status, as well as by the patient's medical need. Thus the patient's social location becomes a variable in determining how his medical condition will be evaluated and handled. Stereotypes of patients that form in the crew culture are used in adjusting the level of patient care. Most of this adjustment is in terms of courtesy and comfort and has little bearing on the patient's health. However, the tendency to underestimate the seriousness of complaints could occasionally lead to significant aggravation of a medical condition.

Thus the patients themselves, along with coworkers, teachers, and employers, help to shape the attendants' activity. There is in addition another set of expectations that directly affects that activity. These expectations are held by the public servants, bystanders, and emergency room personnel with whom the EMT shares responsibility in the care of trauma victims, those with whom the EMTs could be said to have accidental relations.

7

accidental relations

Authority Problems in the Field

> *Listening to your police and fire
> department in action is one of the
> newest and most exciting forms of
> entertainment. It's called "scanning."
> Never before has scanning been so
> much fun and so easy to do.*
> — *from a radio commercial
> for monitoring
> equipment*

People who used to chase ambulances can now arrive ahead of them. Widely available technology makes it possible for these people to receive a dispatch at the same time a crew does and, if they are nearer, to get there first. Rural units making long-distance runs sometimes find an eager scanner already on the scene and trying to be helpful by dragging a victim out of a wrecked automobile. The amount of advertising for monitors indicates that more than a few people have taken up scanning as a hobby.[1] The effects of these sophisticated gadgets illustrate two ways in which the relation of the public to EMS has been changing: (1) they increase public awareness of ambulance services, and (2) they threaten to make the management of the accident scene more difficult.

The Public Eye

The public is in the background of all ambulance work, using the service and paying the bills. Since the mid-1960s the public has been gradually learning more about EMS. Some of the knowledge comes by way of personal accounts of striking experiences.

We parked the ambulance on the infield near a tight turn, where a track official told us the racers might have some problems adjusting on the first few laps. Lyle and Jackie [his girlfriend] and I leaned on the wall and watched the warm-ups. Before long a relative of one of the drivers strolled over and asked if we carried "those paddles" [for defibrillation in cardiac arrest]. I told him we didn't and we wouldn't be allowed to use them anyway. He said, "Well, you can't do me any good then. That's what it takes with me. I was gone once and they used those things on me; got me started again. It was the Riverview paramedics that did it. Yessir. I was gone and here I am walking around."

A surprising number of people today can claim to have been dead, at least briefly, according to clinical definitions. Others speak appreciatively about events they witnessed where the attendants were swift or gentle or effective or courteous. Their stories help to legitimate EMS and to boost the morale of ambulance workers. (At the same time, less flattering stories circulate, too—stories about slow responses or attendants who refused to carry a patient into the hospital until they were paid for the trip.)

As a result of hearing these stories and reading newspaper accounts of individuals who survived because of the quick action of someone who knew how to do cardiopulmonary resuscitation, a growing number of people are learning CPR. Health agencies and even employers are encouraging participation in instruction programs, and some supporters have proposed that CPR training be a required part of college curricula. While it is true that CPR skills deteriorate without practice and that even the trained layman may panic in the face of an emergency, experience with the technique does increase the public's understanding of EMS.

Another way EMS touches the public directly is through the sight and sound of the ambulance. Though the signs that protective services are nearby may comfort some, they irritate others. Complaints about sirens are common and reveal public misunderstandings.[2] State laws, city statutes, and the demands of safety determine for the most part how the sirens are used. For example, the state requires that sirens be used whenever the moving ambulance displays flashing lights. Further, although in Metropolis there are different practices among the private companies on the hospital leg of a run—Wright is thought to use the siren on most runs but CityMed claims to do so less than 10 percent of the time—they are all required by the city to use lights and siren on the way to the scene of a fire department dispatch. Liberty rarely uses the siren on the way to the hospital, and the crews run silent in the alley behind Station 2 because of the neighbors, and sometimes at night (illegally) out of consideration for people sleeping. The tone of the complaints reveals that there is some hostility toward the ambulance services.

Indirect information about EMS comes almost entirely through the media. Stories of lifesaving events and dramatic TV series about rescue squads (for example, "Emergency" and "240-Robert") present a positive picture by emphasizing the heroic aspect of the work. Other media coverage, perhaps the larger part, focuses on the unusual, the shocking, the problematic, and presents a less favorable picture. A typical example was Paul Harvey's national news commentary about a St. Louis ambulance crew that stopped to pick up a pizza while on the way to a hospital with an emergency patient.[3] Also common are media jokes that foster a snickering attitude toward unfamiliar (but useful) techniques. ("They had to fire the Eskimo lifeguard out at the lake; he kept trying to give nose-to-nose resuscitation, and it didn't work.") In Metropolis the leading daily newspaper has run stories about women unsuccessfully trying to become paramedics through the fire department, about delays in ambulance responses for an injured umpire at the stadium and for a disgruntled patron of the Riverside Arts Festival, and about increases in the county-mandated fee for private ambulances. This newspaper gave extensive coverage to a "no transport" who was later discovered to have acute meningitis (see Chapter 6). The original account ran under a five-column headline, the company and crew's defense the next day under a two-column heading, and the eventual exoneration of the crew by the city health department under a one-column lead. The paper's editorial on the case ("How Careful Is Emergency Care?") showed little understanding of local EMS. It underrated the skills of the EMTs, ignored the problem of abuse calls, overlooked the legal constraints on the crew, and unrealistically wondered why a backup physician might not have been consulted. Moreover, the editorial was careful to tell readers where they could call to complain about ambulance services. Support for the EMTs and explanations about the system usually appear only in the letters-to-the-editor columns.

We do not know how knowledge affects the public's attitudes or behavior toward EMS. But just as the circulating information is both favorable and unfavorable, so are the public's responses. The public shows its support of EMS by volunteering time and money, by actively intervening in emergencies, and by training in first aid and CPR. More ambiguous attitudes are evident in the scanners who race to the accident scenes or in the restaurant owners who ask their crew customers to park in back because an ambulance in front might hurt business. Other public behaviors are clearly contemptuous and even antagonistic. Drivers intent on their own purposes might hinder an ambulance even when they are aware of its presence. (Jase would cry out in frustration when a driver cut him off and then hesitated at a light, "Well, what are you waiting for? The pole to turn green?") Crowds sometimes resent being asked to move aside for an ambulance; a stricken spectator died of a heart attack when football players would not allow the ambulance onto the sidelines during a game.[4] Daily, prank callers "cry wolf" and get the operator or dispatcher's adrenalin surging by breathlessly sobbing that they've just been raped or beaten up or that someone is trying to kill them, by mimicking a child who is lost, or by creating the impression of a building in flames ("Fire! Help me, I'm burning!"), before they laugh and hang up or, worse yet, force an ambulance to respond. Though these hostile actions are relatively few, their effect on the system is considerable; they lower morale, waste resources, and sometimes cost lives.

The Definition of a Medical Emergency

The most significant impact the public has on the EMS system is through its typical pattern of use: how people determine when it is appropriate to call an ambulance. We saw in Chapter 6 that people have quite diverse opinions about when an ambulance should be summoned. Even if we disregard the regular nuisance calls, the range of understandings is broad. There seem to be three considerations involved in deciding that a situation is a medical emergency requiring an ambulance: the perception of the medical problem, the perception of the purpose of the ambulance, and the perception of the net cost or benefit to the patient in the light of alternatives.[5]

There is no consensus about which *medical problems* would benefit from an ambulance. Since the attendants sometimes disagree in this regard, it is not surprising that the untrained vary in their judgments. The social characteristics of the definers (usually family or acquaintances) seem to be important; different socioeconomic classes and ethnic groups interpret signs and symptoms differently.[6] The upper classes may, for example, take fainting spells more seriously than do the lower classes (though they do not necessarily treat them as emergencies). Experience is also important in interpreting medical complaints. Those who are familiar with a patient's diabetes or epilepsy respond differently from those who are not. Indeed, to the bystander, any medical problem he feels he cannot cope with is an emergency. Also, the greater the bystander's responsibility for or emotional attachment to the patient, the more likely he is to consider the problem an emergency. Dispatchers, in their screening of calls, assume that family members are more likely to overreact to a medical problem than are other callers. The public's decisions are made more difficult by the fact that the health care system's definition of emergency has been expanding in two directions. On the one hand, emergency rooms have been accepting patients with what were formerly considered minor complaints; on the other hand, cases that were formerly considered hopeless (drownings, cardiac arrests) are now thought of as salvable. It should also be noted here that there is no conclusive link between the definer's thought and his action. Even where conditions are judged to be serious by everyone involved, the behavior sometimes contradicts that judgment. It is not unusual for a family to dress a patient with a suspected back injury or to move someone with a suspected broken hip to a wheelchair, nor is it unheard of for bystanders to treat a broken leg casually or even to drive around looking for a hospital or an ambulance rather than to call one.

How the patient or bystander understands the *purpose of the ambulance* influences his definition of an emergency. If the ambulance provides free transportation to the hospital with no questions asked (as was true in Metropolis when the police provided the service), there is a temptation to designate any medical problem an emergency. Long after a particular service has been reorganized, that simple, old understanding will continue to influence many of the callers. Moreover, where the ambulance is considered to be merely a high-speed bed, which is how many people still see it, there will be less hesitancy to summon it for minor complaints than where it is seen as delivering basic or advanced life support. And for that increasing portion of the population who use the emergency room as their primary care facility,[7] the ambulance is seen as a ministry of the hospital, conveniently making deliveries right to the door. These people are likely to assume that there is a public service to meet any of their needs, and thus to be less self-reliant in dealing with their problems.

Several items enter into what the bystander calculates as the *net cost or benefit* of summoning an ambulance, among them knowledge of a means of access, the probable response time, the financial charge, the threat of a penalty for misuse, and the availability of other means of transportation. If people are not sure how to get in touch with an ambulance (for instance, if the community does not have a 911 emergency number), they will be tempted to do without rather than take the time to find out. The same is true if they think the ambulance will take a long time and they judge the situation to be desperate or want to shed their responsibility for the patient as quickly as possible.[8] A sizable charge for each run or a legal penalty for runs the city finds unnecessary causes definers to hestitate in declaring an emergency. Finally, in some cases emergencies are called for reasons other than medical urgency. The ambulance may be the only means of transportation for a patient who needs care but has no car or no family to help and either cannot get a taxi to come to the house or cannot get into one. With so many variables entering into the public's definition of an emergency, it is no wonder the attendants find little consistency in the urgency of the medical needs they are asked to meet.

The public could be a more positive force in EMS. Citizens could be active collaborators if more learned CPR and first aid and were prepared to use them, and if more became knowledgeable and self-reliant with regard to health. They could at least refrain from calling the ambulance unless it were necessary. The public is hindered in realizing this potential by their fear of legal liability,[9] their tendency to rely on experts, and their old-fashioned ideas about ambulance services. Some of these hindrances might be overcome by public education programs on the Good Samaritan doctrine, on the advantages of self-care, on the meaning of vital signs and certain symptoms, and on the nature and purpose of prehospital EMS. Such programs would not touch the hostile elements within the public or the chronic abusers, but they might alter the prevailing definition of emergency so that the use of the ambulance could more closely match its purpose.

On the Scene

Ambulance work takes place nearly anywhere. Whatever the setting, the attendants can never be concerned with the patient exclusively; inevitably there are others on the scene. There is at least the person who originally summoned the ambulance. Often there are representatives of other public services—police or firefighters—involved as first responders or because of their routine duties. And as soon as the crew departs with the patient, they will probably notify the emergency department of the hospital. Few of the

relations between the people involved in these activities are explicitly defined.[10] Most encounters on the scene go smoothly because of tentative relationships worked out informally through repeated contacts.[11] But a
vagueness remains, because it is impossible to spell out each person's
duties precisely when circumstances are so unpredictable and when for
some participants—the patient and associates—the occasion is extraordinary and unrepeated.

The arrival of emergency medical personnel is like an invasion, especially if the scene is a residence. Maya Angelou evokes the atmosphere in
recalling events from her youth:

*The ambulance screamed as it two-wheel-turned the corner from our
block. I picked Guy up, not noticing his weight, and ran to our house,
where two police cars sat empty, their red eyes turning faintly in the
afternoon sunlight. . . . The sound of police and ambulance sirens
whine through my childhood memories with dateless frequency. The
red lights whirring on top of official cars and the heavy disrespectful
footsteps of strange authority in our houses can be brought back
clearly in my mind at a beckon.*[12]

In the Liberty sector it is not unheard of for the small living room and kitchen of an apartment to contain the patient (possibly a heart attack victim),
two firefighters from the rescue squad, three paramedics, an ambulance
crew of two with an observer along, two neighbors who made the call, and
a relative (also summoned) with spouse and two children, for a total of fifteen people with radios, trauma boxes, oxygen tanks, handbags,
guerneys, and other gear. The event is out of the patient's or family's control, not only because of the number of official intruders, but also because
they do not know how to behave in a medical crisis. Since the normal rules
of conduct are suspended in an emergency, patients have no basis for
judging what is appropriate. They have been known to pretend they were
unconscious until loaded into the ambulance, because they did not know
what was expected of them and so adopted a stereotyped role of the
"ambulance patient."[13] The crews attempt to establish order in the midst of
this uncertainty by imposing their own definition of the situation—that this
is a medical emergency and that they are qualified to handle it. They assert
their right to define the situation by appearing calm, by being active (assessing the patient's condition), and by giving directions (taking charge of
questioning and making arrangements for departure). In most cases the
patient, family, and friends defer to the experience of the crews.

Occasionally other participants override the crew's definition of the
situation.[14] The family, for example, has a large emotional stake in the out-
come of the case because of their concern for the patient's well-being and

their concern (no less potent) about their own responsibility for the patient's predicament. The dread and guilt sometimes issue in tearful remorse ("Oh, my God. How could I have done such a stupid thing?"). At other times they are expressed more aggressively by voice (a woman screamed hysterically at the paramedics who had tried to save her husband, "Do you know how young I am? Do you know how young I am? Do you know?") or by acting out (a frantic daughter tailgated the ambulance all the way to the hospital and then complained that the flashing red light bothered her eyes). The very presence of emotionally demonstrative bystanders may be enough to undermine the attendants' confidence or cause them to take actions they might otherwise avoid. For example, they can be pressured into attempting resuscitation on very old patients. "The doctors tell us to let someone like that go, but if you're called in and grandpa's stopped breathing, you can't just say, 'Let him die'." Emergency room personnel, too, occasionally complain about the interference of the patient's friends and acquaintances.

Families that are fragmented or that consist of tenuous relationships cause different problems. The crews have to determine who can give permission to move an incapacitated person or minor and who will be responsible for paying. Therefore they must decide whether the "aunt" in the house is a genuine relative, or whether it is appropriate to have the live-in "friend" sign the trip slip. Perhaps before leaving for the hospital the crew will have to arrange for temporary disposition of the children or inquire about billing the run to a separated and hostile spouse.

People on the scene who are not directly involved are referred to as *bystanders,* though there are different kinds. The crews speak with disdain of "rubberneckers," who go out of their way to look at an accident; they are more neutral about "onlookers," who happen to be nearby and are curious. Bystanders might also be people who lend a hand in the emergency by telephoning for the ambulance, holding a bandage, or helping with the gurney. The crews are wary of bystanders, even though they sometimes provide useful information or assist in other ways. The crews make it a rule to close all the doors when they leave the ambulance to reduce the temptation for the crowd to explore it or even to steal equipment. A subcategory of the helpful bystander is the intervenor, a physician who happens on the scene and decides to take charge, although his presence has not been specifically requested.[15] Because of his training and status, the physician often feels obliged to assert himself, even though he may be less skilled in basic emergency procedures (such as CPR) than the ambulance personnel.[16] The EMTs tell stories about the physician who leaped to begin CPR and immediately broke several of the patient's ribs, and the attendant who shouted at a stranger, a physician, who was rotating a patient's ankle, which was possibly broken. Physician intervention creates more serious conflicts for the paramedics, because they have their own protocols to follow and their own delegated medical authority.[17] The basic EMT is probably more likely to defer to the physician. In both cases there is the problem of establishing whether a stranger who presents himself as a physician is legitimate; in an emergency there is no time for checking credentials. The behavior of the family and of bystanders is one of the unpredictable features of ambulance work.

The other people the crews regularly see on the scene are the first responders. The first official to arrive is usually a law enforcement agent (policeman or sheriff's deputy) or a firefighter. In Metropolis the fire department responds first to most medical emergencies, although certain calls originate with the police, and in certain cases the private ambulances go in alone. Individual attendants have personal friendships and animosities with members of the other services, as one would expect, but the ambulance crews also share an attitude toward the other services that is related to the structure of their own work. Because their missions are different, the police and ambulance crews are complementary and therefore somewhat alien; the police are not much interested in medical services.[18] The firefighters share a mission (patient care) with the crews and a common outlook with those attendants who also serve as volunteer firefighters, but this similarity often turns into competition.

The primary concerns of the *police* on the scene are to maintain public safety and to gather evidence. In the interest of public safety, the police at an accident may give priority to getting the roadway cleared and traffic moving. This aim is in conflict with that of the EMT, who wants to do a careful assessment and extrication of the patient. Or the EMT may disagree with the sheriff's mounted patrol about whether a particular victim should be treated with CPR ("I'm sure I saw that one moving. You guys better do something.") Few police are trained in basic life support.[19] When differences occur, the policeman has a badge and a gun to back up his opinion, while the attendant must rely on persuasion to make his point. As one EMT put it when asked what he liked about doing rescue squad work with a police department, "Well, for one thing I don't have any problems of authority."

In gathering evidence, the police like to have the cooperation of the attendants. This normally requires no more from the EMTs than giving the patient's name and address. Now and then they might be asked about the position or condition of a victim, or the investigations unit at the hospital might want some background on an attempted suicide, or on rare occasions EMTs might be required to serve as witnesses in court (see below). Here, too, there is a possibility of conflict. The police want to use the crews to accomplish police business. In Metropolis the chief of police tried to retain control of EMS on the grounds that valuable evidence could be gathered in the ambulance. The EMTs, however, feel that they can do their job only if the patient is able to assume a degree of confidentiality in their relationship. On one run an attendant worked for fifteen minutes to persuade an OD (drug overdose) to turn over a sample of the street drugs he had taken; the patient would have been even more worried about self-incrimination if the attendant had been a policeman. Further, patrolmen and attendants sometimes disagree about what evidence is pertinent.

Skip was telling about an encounter with the police. His crew had found a woman DOE on a bed. There was a large stain of dried blood on the floor of the room but none between the spot and the bed. The face was livid [discolored from the pooling of blood] on the upper side as the body lay there. The patrolman suggested that she had "bled out" while standing and then fell onto the bed. Skip pointed out that the explanation didn't account for the lividity, but the cop didn't want to deal with that evidence. It would mean he would have to make out a raft of reports. B.Z. said in such cases it is OK to call the Bureau of Detectives directly; they would be grateful. He said the patrolmen are reluctant to take steps that will require more work of them.

Different perspectives on the relative importance of medical care and safety and on the uses of patient information insure at least a modest tension between the personnel of these two services.[20]

In the Liberty sector the privates and the police maintain calm if not cordial relations. The attendants share information with the police and take many drunks off their hands. For their part, the police provide protection for the crews (at Gino's Bar, for example), rescue them when necessary (Flash, Louie, Jardine, and Jase, among others, have benefited from their help), and occasionally pass along a compliment ("You guys know what to do pretty fast when you get here.") Still, the attendants' reservations are evident in Tanner's surprise when he saw a squad car block off a cross-street to clear the way for the ambulance running hot: "Look at that! They're actually giving us a hand. I can't believe it!"

There are several reasons for the crews' irritation with the police. First, they assume the police are keeping an eye on them. Rumors circulate that the police will contact the company base to try to catch crews using the red lights and siren unnecessarily. Word was that a Towner driver had been ticketed for running hot to take two friends home. The attendants also hesitate to look in a patient's purse or wallet for information, because they feel the police already suspect them of stealing; in return, they joke about how a DOE's wallet never contains cash after the police have checked it. Second, they resent the police wanting them to haul drunks and bums who could as easily be transported by squad car or paddywagon. The police are angry about the crews' reluctance: "Don't complain so much. We gave the last three [drunks] to Wright [Ambulance Service]. . . . Why the hell did the city give you the contract [to transport medical emergencies] if you don't haul anyone all day?" Once it was decided that the city had to bear the costs of ambulance runs initiated by the police, and once the senior officers informed the troops that they were not to give incapacitation papers (which established the city's liability) for hauling drunks, the number of calls from the police declined noticeably. Third, runs to the "cop shop" (district headquarters and lock-up) are almost always for minor problems—bruises and lacerations—but are inaccurately presented as emergencies (to get the rigs there more quickly, it is suspected).

Jardine is angry about our not getting better information from the police on a dispatch. He feels it is stupid and unproductive to run hot for a case where there is no threat to life. Even a fractured ankle, for example, is not going to get significantly worse in a few more minutes. But the danger of driving fast in traffic is a serious matter. Jardine talked about having such close shaves while driving hot that he was nervous for a long while after.

Following the owner's complaint to the police, runs to the cop shop were 10-16 (respond immediately without lights and siren) for about a week. However, supposedly because of communication problems between the police and the fire department dispatchers, the requests for silent running were lost, and soon the minor ailments reverted to emergency status. Fourth, it is difficult to get the police to comply with regulations. Although they are required to provide papers for any patient they designate as incapacitated (unable to give informed consent) and to accompany the patient in the ambulance, they are reluctant to do either. Even when they want to MO (institutionalize for mental observation) a patient who is considered a danger to himself (for example, an attempted suicide), they try to avoid filling out an emergency detention form by pressuring the crew to take him as a voluntary admission. Sometimes their "forgetting" covers blatant deception—"We don't have any forms in the squad, but you go on out to County and we'll pick them up and meet you there."

Part of the antagonism between the crews and the police grows out of authority differences and part out of the different understandings of emergency care. Friction is also generated by each service's effort to make its job as easy as possible. As Roth put it, employees "are concerned with applying a set of rules which will keep their work demands within bounds and will keep them out of trouble with their superiors."[21] They do this by establishing routines that will shift as much of the work load as possible onto other services. For the police, this means minimizing public complaints about sirens, getting rid of drunks and bums and minor injuries quickly, and avoiding paperwork. For the crews, it means letting the police hassle drunks and psychos, avoiding dangerous trips through traffic, and using police paper whenever possible. Each service pursues its self-interest toward eventual accommodation. In Metropolis the common understanding is still being worked out.

The crews in Metropolis are in contact with *firefighters* on every emergency run, because the calls come through the fire department dispatcher. In addition, the ambulances are usually preceded on the scene by a fire department rescue squad or engine company. One might expect the steady contact and shared mission to lead to friendly relations, and indeed there are some warm acquaintances between individuals in the two services. However, the general feelings of the attendants toward fire department personnel are competitive and critical. These feelings seem to be related to problems of authority, relative deprivation, and responsibility.

The fire department dispatcher, who controls the crews' lives without being subject to their advice or consent, is a constant reminder that the company is a dependent operation. This condition is particularly galliing when the ambulances are blamed for slow responses even though the crews are sure they have made a fast run. The attendants point out that the delays in several publicized cases were due to a breakdown in communications. The loss of time seems to be especially noticeable when dispatching and responding are handled by different agencies, and the problem is not limited to Metropolis. An attendant for a private company in another city questioned a visiting lecturer about a similar difficulty:

EMT: *Why does the police dispatcher give a ten-fifty PI [personal injury] and then wait until the cruiser is on the scene before the ambulance is called? It happens nine times out of ten. I listen on a monitor down at the base. The cruiser says, "Is that ten-fifty-two [ambulance] enroute?" And the dispatcher says, "Yes." And then the phone rings.*
POLICE OFFICER: *Well, that's bad. I've been faulting you guys when you're not to blame. I'll bring that up at the station. I will.*

In the field the crews are technically under the authority of the firefighters, though they can usually manage their patients without interference. For the most part the Liberty EMTs are ignored by the paramedics, whose condescension seems to be used equally on everyone and is dismissed as resulting from their temporary self-images as "Junior Jehovahs." The crews *are* bothered by people they know who, since they have become paramedics, are "too good" to associate with lowly EMTs.

The crews recognize that firefighters have the authority but question whether they are worthy of it. They see the fire department as having too narrow a view of the EMS system. Jardine expressed this criticism in a meeting with the commissioner of health:

The mobile units are trained to work on their own under a physician's direction; they are not ready to control a disaster scene or even to do triage [classify victims by seriousness of injury]. The night of the fire at the Avenue Motel there were twenty-two patients transported. They only requested one ambulance; we sent three and they used them all. They told everyone to take the patients to St. Christopher. Fortunately the hospital was changing shifts at the time so there was plenty of personnel. But a lot of the cases were fractures caused by jumping from the second story. The St. Chris staff asked why they weren't taken to St. Jude, which has a specialty in orthopedics. Liberty conveyed three patients who went into the hyperbaric [pressure] chamber. Who did the mobiles carry? Heart patients with no symptoms!

Even in less extraordinary situations the fire department does not coordinate well with other services. Occasionally the rescue squads take vitals but forget to pass them along to the private crews that transport the patients; the paramedics rarely volunteer information on their cases. The attendants claim that typically the mobile units leave nothing behind but the body and the promise that an ambulance will pick it up. The privates arrive to find a DOE with the paramedics' intravenous catheters still in place, the family hysterical, and no history or other information on the patient. The emergency room staff are furious at having a body dropped on them with no information.[22] In one case it was a three-month-old, the body blue and obvious injuries on the head. In spite of the commissioner of health's admitting the need for better liaison among the components of the EMS system, there have been no significant changes in operations. Some of the crews believe the reason is that the fire department does not have a full-time administrator assigned to EMS; one of the officials oversees it in addition to his regular duties.

Since they are doing essentially the same work, the firefighters' greater authority, pay, and prospects irritate the attendants. Complaints about the injustice of the situation are common in the crew culture. One of the ways the attendants deal with their feelings of relative deprivation is by rewarding themselves with evidence of their superior skills or, more often, evidence of the firefighters' inferior skills. Stories are told about the ignorance of the squad members: they do not splint properly; they do not appreciate the extent of injuries; they sometimes use high-flow oxygen for emphysema victims; they do not know why a humidifier is on the oxygen supply; they cut the knees out of trousers to get at cuts rather than lift the pant legs; they do a sling-and-swathe by wrapping the chest with a bandage and adding a sling. There are grumblings about the fire department sending engine companies to medical emergencies simply to insure a good response time for the department's records and in spite of the fact that there are rarely competent EMTs on the engines. Sal complains about this in particular:

The woman was lying there on the public street and this [fire depart-ment] captain pulls a blanket over her. He says she's dead, take her away. I checked for a radial pulse and it was weak but it was there. I shook her and she started breathing. [exaggerating] A save! A save! I revived her! We put her on the cot and took off. She coded on the way to the hospital; we started CPR. They worked on her at the hospital for about forty minutes. She didn't make it. But maybe if the Fire Depart-ent had . . . [shrugs].

The competitive feelings of the crews grow into an adversary relation-ship in which they see themselves as exercising a kind of quality control over the firefighters. Indeed the owner of Wright Ambulance Service once said the commissioner of health had asked the privates to keep an eye on the rescue squads. (Contrarily, Anderson, who teaches EMT classes, says the EMS system was put in the hands of the fire department because the privates will do anything for profit and because there is better quality con-trol through a public agency. He also admits that many of the firefighters who work as EMTs are forced to do so and thus are not committed to the work.) One of the most striking stories about quality concerns a mobile unit:

10:30 PM. We are sitting in quarters talking about the paramedics. The Doctor says he heard that St. Christopher is going to file a com-plaint about the paramedics' treatment of the code he and Flash had last Saturday. "But they're Kardijan's [medical director of County Hospital's emergency department] babies, so I guess nothing will happen. But it's nice to have even that amount of support." I ask him to tell me the story but he's reluctant. Then Flash says, "OK. You want to hear the story, I'll tell you the story." He says he and The Doctor got a fire call. It was a simultaneous response with Squad 18 and Mobile 2. Liberty got to the scene first. The family ran out to flag them down. The patient (21 yo w/f) was lying on the grass in the yard. She was un-responsive and was red-purple blotchy along the face and arm of one side. Evidently she had been in the garage with the motor running. Possible carbon monoxide [CO] poisoning. (The respiratory therapist from County told us it takes an hour and twenty minutes to reduce the CO attached to the hemoglobin from 20 percent down to 10 percent, and an additional period of the same length to reduce it to 5 percent.)

The Doctor said there was some stiffness in the body but he didn't
think it was rigor mortis. The Doctor said he got both a carotid pulse
(but only on one side) and a radial pulse. The patient's breathing was
shallow or arrested. They began to bag [give artificial respiration].
The Doctor said he had a good airway; the chest was rising when he
bagged. Then Mobile 2 arrived. They started to set an IV and then
wanted to intubate [run a tube from the mouth through the throat
directly to the lungs]. It took them four tries to get the ET [endo-
tracheal] tube in. They never did get the IV going. By the time they got
the heart monitor attached (after having interrupted the resuscitation
efforts), the patient was showing a straight line [no heart activity]. The
Doctor is sure the patient was still alive when they got there. He is
angry that Mobile 2 disregarded the airway they already had and took
too long to reopen it. He and Flash thought the best procedure would
be to transport with CPR to the hyperbaric chamber at St. Christo-
pher. There they could have reduced the CO concentration more
quickly. The event reinforced their opinion that the paramedics are
too rigidly wedded to a set of procedures and therefore don't treat the
individual case in the most promising way.[23]

This adversary posture comes close to hostility at times. Jardine tacked up
a cartoon that showed an ambulance, which he labeled "Death Two," and
a victim's body, on which he recorded each code Mobile 2 failed to save.
He suggested that morgues in the hospitals be called "paramedic rooms."
Other attendants would point out a particular fire station as the base of
"Death Two."

The crews not only complain about the fire department, they take a defensive stance. Rookies are warned always to indicate on their reports if
data, diagnosis, or treatment have come from the fire department, so
Liberty will not be held responsible for the fire department's mistakes. This
includes noting what is *not* done—a patient moved without a spineboard,
for example. As Jardine would say, "The name of the game is CYA
—cover your ass."

The evidence used by the crews in their judgments about the fire department is anecdotal and therefore not an adequate basis for evaluation. Nor
are the crew's observations consistent. At one time they say the low quality
of the rescue squads is a result of the best having been taken for the paramedics; another time they criticize the paramedics for not recruiting good
EMTs. What they see are people they feel are no more competent than
themselves moving up, while they do not have the same opportunities.
Whether the evaluations are accurate is not as important for the crews' behavior as the fact that they are believed. It is the belief that leads to com-
petitiveness, adversary relations, and even hostility. The importance of the

firefighters' relative status in stimulating these feelings can be seen in the fact that the attendants do not display the same attitudes toward the other private ambulance companies. With the exception of two groups, Happy Harry's Health Hut, which provides volunteer first aid at rock concerts ("They're irresponsible fuck-offs. They don't know what they're doing. They've been kicked out of the Riverside Arts Festival."), and one of the privates (Tanner pointed to a hearse in the traffic. "Isn't that one of Towner's new ambulances?"), relations among the privates are fairly cordial. It appears that criticisms of the fire department help to build cohesion among the ambulance workers, who do not have so many advantages.

At the Hospital

The prehospital phase of emergency medical care ends in the emergency department. Whether the end of a particular run is smooth or abrupt depends on the crew's relationships with the ED staff. Where emergency medical services are not closely regulated, the differences among EDs can be significant. The Liberty crews have to comply with the preferences of individual hospitals, even in radio communications. One ED wants to be notified of every incoming patient; another wants advance warning only if the patient requires a bed; another wants to hear only about critical patients; another rarely answers radio calls, and the crews sometimes resort to having their dispatcher telephone that hospital. At St. Christopher's Hospital the expectations about radio calls change from shift to shift.

The lack of coordination of radio communications accurately indicates the quality of overall EMS regulation in Metropolis. Each organization in the EMS system operates as an independent entity (which indeed it is) and negotiates mutually acceptable work routines with other participating organizations. The interests of the system as a whole get little attention. St. John's Hospital has put considerable effort into its own plan for handling future disasters but assumes that coordination will not be a problem in a mass emergency. The hospital has not consulted the ambulance companies about patterns of ambulance movement, traffic control, availability of gurneys for off-loading patients, a system of victim identification, or many other difficulties that attend medical catastrophe. The consequences of a fragmented EMS system range from small savings to large misunderstandings, and all of them affect patient care. At the very least, fragmentation causes inefficiencies. The electrode pads a hospital attaches to a heart patient, for example, do not fit the leads to Liberty's heart monitor. More important, since each organization follows its own preferences, there can be no equipment exchange among the hospitals and the ambulances. If an ambulance delivers a patient with a traction splint attached, it cannot take a replacement splint from the hospital but must run without until it returns to pick up its own. To be sure, it is not only the EMS organizations that show problems of coordination. There are similar disjunctions between ambulance companies and nursing homes. For instance, when they have a patient transferred to a hospital, the nursing homes routinely seal the patient's records in an envelope. The attendants, who need some of the information for their reports, routinely open the envelope in the ambulance and copy what they want. Since the hospitals do not complain about the torn envelopes and the nursing homes do not know about them, everyone seems to be happy with the arrangement.[24] Thus it is not the *emergency* aspect alone that undermines orderly cooperation.

Moreover, there are problems of coordination inside organizations, as well as between them. Information gets lost or distorted when it is moved from one unit to another. It is not unusual for official records to include misspelled names; the name on one nursing home patient's nightstand did not agree with the name on either of two forms attached to her records. Communication problems also arise between authority levels within a unit—St. Christopher's ED staff could not get adequate support until they maneuvered the nursing supervisor into working a Saturday night shift and experiencing the problems firsthand. Even the discontinuities in tasks occasioned by a worker's attempt to satisfy too many demands reduce the efficiency of patient care. When the ED nurse lays down an unmarked envelope of street drugs to attend to an important request, will she later remember where the envelope is, what it contains, and what patient it is connected with?

The crews are outranked by the ED personnel, who in most cases can give them directions. The most obvious example of ED control is the "bypass alert,"[25] which notifies the ambulances that the hospital has no room for additional emergency patients. St. Christopher imposes such bans once or twice a week.[26] (The crews are able to express a small degree of independence by occasionally delivering a messy drunk, whom the ED staff cannot refuse.) In most matters the crews and the patients have little basis for successfully challenging the staff's decisions. Clark described a typical disagreement:

The Sexual Abuse Treatment Team at Friendship [Hospital] wouldn't take a rape case on Friday night. They say they can't take a minor without a parent's consent or a patient who has any trauma [physical injury]. We were there with a thirteen-year-old. [With heavy irony.] She had major trauma. There were some scratches on her arms! The nurse was ready to take her. We talked her into it. Then the team supervisor said "No." So we stood there in the hall and argued about it. How's that for a fine community resource?

Not only must the crews accept directions from the EDs, they realize they must do it respectfully, even though that respect is not always reciprocated. As one EMT expressed it, the EMTs understand "they are part of the medical community only so long as they maintain enough deference not to threaten the R.N.s, physicians, and hospital administrators. . . ."[27] Another said he is treated with respect during the week, when he works in the hospital as a clinic administrator, but on the weekends, when he serves as an EMT, he is addressed by the nurses as "boy," "gurney lifter," or "driver."[28] This lack of respect is implied in the common complaint of ambulance workers that ED personnel disregard their reports and recheck everything they have done.[29] Under these conditions perhaps it should be no surprise that the attendants try to assert themselves in ways that are not necessarily appropriate. Among the Liberty attendants, Van Buskirk was noted for his righteous disrespect. He riled an ED supervisor by recording his opinion of a female patient on the EMT report using the very personal (but rather dated) phrase, "Hubba-hubba."

Van Buskirk once corrected an MD about the exact nature of a drug. The MD disagreed and Van Buskirk pulled out a supplement to the PDR [Physician's Desk Reference] to prove his point. Van Buskirk was right, but the MD was so angry that he called the company to complain. It was this sort of behavior that led to Van Buskirk's being fired, according to Jase.

The attitudes of the ED people toward the Liberty EMTs are probably influenced by the fact that they work for a private company. The nurses who have been around for even a few years remember a time when the privates competed shamelessly for business from the hospitals. The passing out of gifts (pens, cups, calendars) was so constant the ED staff would greet the attendants by asking, "What did you bring us today?" One ED staff member called to ask if Liberty would pick up a pizza for them, to which (so the story goes) an indignant Harold replied, "Wait a minute! I think you misunderstand the business we're in." Although circumstances have altered and now the hospitals are trying to encourage more business, the ED people still seem to have reservations about the private ambulances' interest in profit. The staff disapproval is apparent (in frowns and head shaking) when the attendants attempt to reach a financial settlement before taking a patient out of the hospital. If the settlement is not satisfactory, the attendants may ask the hospital to take responsibility for the costs before they move the patient. The ambulance workers are caught in the middle between the hospital and the company. Further, the ED staffs show they are suspicious of the attendants when they closely screen their requests for replacement of expendable equipment. It is not clear whether the hospital personnel are aware that attendants also sneak extra supplies from the storerooms.[30]

The attendants have more contact with the nurses in the ED than with the physicians, so they complain more about the nurses. This pattern is not peculiar to Metropolis; a lot has been written about conflict between ED nurses and paramedics or EMTs. The trouble has been attributed to nurses being rigidly committed to traditional patterns, being defensive because they feel their jobs are threatened, and being uncertain about what their role should be in the EMS system.[31] (On the other side, the paramedics and EMTs are charged with uncritically going for the latest fads, being generally insensitive, and acting like know-it-alls.) Of course, their different institutional loyalties probably also contribute to the difficulties between nurses and EMTs. All these factors are important in creating conflict. But surely a great deal can be explained by the fact that the two parties have different goals and different procedures. Because of their different goals, they give priorities to distinct tasks. Anderson, the EMT instructor, said ED nurses complain to him that they cannot get a good blood-gas (laboratory test) if the ambulance crew has loaded the patient with oxygen. Anderson said he simply disregards them, because if it were not for the oxygen, they probably wouldn't have a live patient to do tests on. From time to time the nurses want to do a procedure (a blood sample, for example) while the patient is still on Liberty's guerney, or the physicians go to work without moving the patient to a bed. The attendants usually resent these presumptions because, while they show a commendable preoccupation on the part of the hospital staff, they also show a disregard for the mission of the ambulance workers, who are expected to clear promptly and get back in service.

The Liberty attendants complain loudest about the ED staff's procedures, which they interpret as showing a lack of knowledge.[32] These complaints are sometimes affected by personal relationships (varying from intense romances to unrelenting antagonism) between EMTs and ED personnel. Cynthia, who is in charge of one of the shifts at the Zion ED, was a friend of the crews for a long time, but after a disagreement, she became the subject of a whole catalog of complaints. However, the nature and distribution of complaints about ED nurses suggest they are more than petty insults. The attendants complain that ED nurses remove traction splints and spineboards before the patients have been X-rayed for fractures (one X-ray technician did not know what a traction splint was), that they have not heard of giving glucose to an unconscious diabetic, that they do not know you should cover both eyes to prevent movement even if only one is injured, that in some circumstances you can give an emphysema patient more than a two-liter flow of oxygen, that carbon monoxide is odorless ("Oh, I can smell the carbon monoxide on him."), and that you need all those straps to immobilize a patient adequately ("We never had all this stuff when the police were running the ambulances.").[33] The EMTs are even in-structed at in-service workshops to lean over the patient on the guerney so the ED staff cannot attempt to remove the MAST (Medical Anti-Shock Trousers) devices until the implications of deflating them can be fully ex-plained.

The different understandings of what should be done make communica-tion more difficult. The staff hears what it expects to hear. When Gundy handed over an infant whose finger tip had been torn off, the physician thought he said "convulsion" rather than "avulsion." In many cases ED personnel simply do not listen, because they feel there is nothing they can learn from the crews.

The receptionist at Friendship [Hospital] told us to take the patient straight up to the ward. While we were transferring him onto the bed, The Doctor told the nurse in charge that the patient was in a phase of Cheyne-Stokes breathing [alternating periods of rapid respiration and no respiration]. We had just pushed the guerney into the hall when someone shouted, "He's arrested! Call the cart!" We looked into the room and saw the nurse up on the bed on her knees starting to do CPR on the patient we had just transported. We were pushed aside by someone rushing into the room and there was a clatter behind us as others arrived with the resuscitation cart. One of the new arrivals said, "He's breathing!" The frantic activity stopped and the crowd watched the patient intently. The Doctor and I looked at each other. "A save?" I asked.

The misunderstanding and miscommunication between the crews and the ED personnel seem to be largely a result of different experiences and different training. From the EMT's perspective, the EDs do not appreciate what work in the field is like and therefore make unrealistic demands of the ambulance workers. An ED physician recognized the disjunction between his role and that of the paramedics: ". . . the physician gives an order to intubate, is in a position to continue with care of the intubated patient, but is not trained in intubation himself!"[34] In order to increase the experience of the people with whom they have to cooperate, the Liberty crews are usually happy to have front office and hospital personnel ride with them, but it only happens once or twice a month. An ED nurse from Phoenix re-ported, "When we started to put the nurses out on the streets to ride along, the antagonistic ones fell by the wayside. They found out they weren't as smart as they thought they were."[35] Even though the nurses get special in-struction for emergency department duty, the instruction comes through the hospital rather than through the EMS system. One ED nurse in Metro-polis, who trained as an EMT, said she couldn't believe how different it was from what she had learned before. She claimed that some of the things they were taught to do on emergency service as nurses were simply wrong.

Unfortunately the different views of the two services are not reconciled by formal conversations between them. There are no institutionalized procedures for mutual evaluation of the EMTs and the ED personnel in Metropolis, although such arrangements are routine in other places. The ED nurses are most likely to ignore the Liberty attendants; occasionally they will make a critical comment, and only rarely will they compliment someone, perhaps about a clear and concise radio transmission.[36] At the least, the several components of an EMS system need to have some common training (and therefore establish some shared knowledge) and participate in each other's work setting in order to develop role empathy (and thus more realistic expectations).[37] These steps toward better coordination of activities could be taken without altering the present organizational affiliations of the participants. However, the fact that the firefighters and the privates are in conflict, even though they already train together and understand each other's roles, indicates that more extensive organizational changes might be necessary for a fully integrated system.

In the Courts

Ambulance workers are likely to be summoned to appear in court because they have direct knowledge of accidents and injuries, some of which may involve criminal action. In such cases the crews' testimony and records are subject to public scrutiny. The attendant can be under considerable pressure, and an awareness of the sources will tell him a lot about the criminal justice system and about himself. Flash and I were involved in a case that illustrates these points.

One evening a deputy sheriff delivered to my home a subpoena requiring me to appear in court. He said he had no idea what the case was about. Since the document had initially been delivered to me at the Liberty Ambulance address, I called the company to see what they knew about it. Helen in the front office said that Flash had been subpoenaed also, that we were to appear as witnesses, and that she would send me copies of the trip slip and EMT report for the run they were interested in. The trial was called for December 12th and concerned a patient we had handled on July 9th. The report mentioned some bruises and lacerations on the face of our patient and listed the cause of injury as "alleged assault." My field notes did not add much to that account.

8:45 PM. Immediately we got a fire call. Went hot down Frankford and across Oak, over to 16th and down to Fern. There was a crowd of people in front of the house, and the MFD had an engine and squad on

*the scene. The patient was inside lying face down on a bed. He thought
he could walk to the rig but had to get his sandals on his bare feet first.
Wardell Brown. About 35 y.o. B/M. [Actually 42 y.o.] Said he had
been jumped and beaten up. Had lacerations on his head. We took
him to Zion. Flash said he [the patient] could register himself, so he
pushed the wheelchair [standard for somewhat unsteady patients] up
to the admitting desk. Flash went into the lounge to see what was
happening there. We cleared at 9:21 PM.*

At the courthouse on the day of the trial, we learned that our patient was
charging another man with assault. Flash talked to some policemen he
knew while we were all waiting.

*Flash comes back with a pair of color photos of the injured party with
white patch bandages over one eye, under the other, and on his chin.
Flash points out that I hadn't mentioned the chin in my EMT report. I
have a vague recollection of the patient but am not sure he was really
the one we had treated. Flash says he recognizes the guy with no
trouble.*

*The assistant district attorney who is handling the case introduces
himself and sits down with us. He compliments the policemen for taking the photos; considers it good work. I ask what he wants from us.
He says just to demonstrate his client was at the address and was injured. I ask what if I'm not sure the party is the one we carried? He
says, "Oh, you won't have any trouble recognizing him. He has a very
distinctive appearance." I think he was commenting about my match-
ing the photos with the actual person, but I meant I could not be sure
who it was we conveyed on that occasion. He couldn't see how I could
not remember, and passed over the whole matter.*

I noted in Chapter 5 that the patients begin to blur together for ambulance workers. Unless an event is especially vivid for some reason (and this
one was not) or the individual is strikingly peculiar in some respect (and
this one was not), it is not likely that an attendant would be able to distinguish a face seen once six months before from hundreds of others seen in a
similar context before and after.

*I begin to feel pressure to say I can remember even when I'm not sure.
Flash seems to be very certain. The DA has no doubts. The police are
used to this. But I am unsure.*

Since we were available, the DA pulled out some medical records on
Brown and asked us if we could make anything of them. The most im-

pressive fact for me was the disparity between the reports from different sources. Most were poorly written, the terminology was not consistent, there were three versions of the name, and the birth dates and expressed ages did not match. Moreover, there was no evidence that any of the medical care providers knew of the treatments given by the others.

I show Flash the page from my research notes that includes our picking up Brown. He says, "Oh, yeah, I remember that evening." Does he really? He reads on and gets some chuckles from my comments about other matters on the page. Some black men move into the courtroom and sit down. They go out again. Flash says, "That's the guy that got hit." I say I remembered him as more slender. This guy is short and stocky. The black guys come back. Flash says, "Yeah, that's him."

I start to decide to agree that this is the guy. I guess it's to help sustain a picture of reality that others are so sure of. Perhaps my ego is too weak. At any rate Flash is sure and I am not. But I am leaning toward taking his word for it. I'm starting to make up my mind to lie. Actually, it is the defendant who looks familiar to me rather than this other guy.

After a conversation between the lawyers and judge, the case is "dismissed without prejudice." Someone mistakenly told the other witnesses and the plaintiff they didn't have to come in today. This circumstance means Brown was not present. So Flash was wrong in "recognizing" him. And I was right in my doubts. I guess I felt I should recognize the patient. I do remember some faces: Dagmar Lafferty (a regular), Wollenkraft (who wanted to die), etc., but not all. So it's not remarkable that this is one I wouldn't remember. But there seems to be a conviction that I should remember.

The DA was furious about the mix-up and said he would reopen the case. He told us he would need only one of us as a witness. Flash volunteered, since the company would pay him while he was in court. I was not eager to return.

This case shows how the EMT plays a small part in events that have wider ramifications. And it shows how the individual can be caught up in the social drama and be subtly coerced into meeting the dominant expectations and supporting the dominant patterns of behavior. In an analogous way, the EMTs are manipulated by remote authorities whose decisions shape the way ambulance work is carried out. While the crews concern themselves with the essentials of daily duties, their world is altered by the politics of emergency care.

the politics of emergency care

The Ambulance in a Larger Setting

MEETING AGENDA
METROPOLITAN COUNTY COUNCIL
ON EMERGENCY MEDICAL SERVICES

Date: October 25, 1979
Time: 1:00 PM
Location: Courthouse Annex, Assembly Room
I.   Roll call
II.   Approval of minutes of September 27, 1979, meeting
III.   New business:
            — Nominating committee report
            — Report on emergency information kits for the elderly
            — Feasibility of paramedic service — southern zone
            — Paramedic program audit report
            — Paramedic area report
IV.   Old business
V.   Committee reports
VI.   Staff report
VII.   Date and time of next meeting
VIII.   Adjournment

Please call 516-6762 by October 24, 1979, if you cannot attend.

Few of the Liberty EMTs have ever heard of the Metropolitan County Council on Emergency Medical Services (MCCEMS). It is never mentioned in quarters, to my knowledge, and the one time it was referred to at an in-service meeting in my hearing the name was garbled. The crews do not have much interest in the government and quasi-government agencies that claim authority over them, nor in the professional and semi-professional associations that claim to promote their interests. Yet these agencies and associations to a large extent shape the work lives of the EMTs.

Where the Action Was

For Metropolis it was the MCCEMS that exercised the most power during the formative stages of the local EMS system. It received funds from federal agencies, advice from the state, cooperation from the regional Health Systems Agency, and the attention of all the influential people interested in emergency care. The County Council, or something like it, was necessary because federal legislation (see Chapter 1) required the general improvement of emergency medical services, and state legislation gave specific conditions for that improvement. When the members of the council first took their seats in 1975, the city of Metropolis was receiving public ambulance transportation from the police department, whose officers, according to state regulations, would have to be retrained by 1978 and whose ambulances would have to be replaced by 1979. While Liberty and the other private companies had begun to do their regular hiring and purchasing with the new regulations in mind, the city was faced with making systemwide alterations. The suburban areas within the county were also looking for ways to satisfy the new regulations economically. Local planning had begun in 1972, when the mayor of Metropolis appointed a six-member advisory group called the Urban EMS Council, which applied for a grant from the Robert Wood Johnson Foundation. The Urban Council became inoperative in 1974, when its funds ran out, but it left behind a set of recommendations, including the establishment of a countywide paramedic program and a single emergency telephone number (911). Interested persons looked for a successor group that would be extensive enough to encompass all affected parties and that could provide the financial support and the legislative power needed to accomplish something. The county government which was implied in the Urban Council's recommendations seemed to satisfy these requirements, and there was enough agreement to allow for the formation of MCCEMS.

The County Council had twenty-one members selected to represent most of the institutions with an interest in EMS.[1] The organizations included at least the following:

private ambulance companies (9);
fire departments (14);
police departments (6);
municipal governments (19);
the Metropolitan County Board of Supervisors;
the State Division of Health;
the Comprehensive Health Planning Agency of the East Central Region;
the Prudential College of Medicine;
the Metropolitan County Medical Society;
Vo-Tech, the state-sponsored, two-year technical college (2 branches);
hospitals (21);
emergency rooms (14);
the State EMTs' Association;
the District Nurses' Association.

Each of the organizations had its own understanding of what was necessary, and each had its own interest to protect. Certainly the components
were in no sense a coordinated EMS system. Officially, the attendants
were represented (though none of them knew it) by a Metropolis resident
named Fairfield, who was a member of the State EMTs' Association. However, none of the Liberty EMTs had ever heard of him; and the council
rarely heard *from* him, since he was silent at all the meetings I attended.
The meetings were dominated by several physicians who had been active
in emergency medical work and, when questions of finance came up, by
representatives of municipal governments.

While the Liberty attendants were making routine transfers and passing
out coffee mugs bearing the company logo, the County Council was making decisions that would affect the EMTs' careers. Three concerns emerged
repeatedly in their deliberations: the need for political support, the difficulty of securing finances, and the problems of control over field operations. A decision in one area of concern affected each of the others, and
each decision affected the prospects of local ambulance workers.

Political support was important, because unless the several municipalities accepted whatever EMS plan was put forward, it would not be passed
by the County Board of Supervisors. The council members wanted their
efforts to result in action and therefore favored solutions with the least potential for political backlash. It was evident early in the deliberations that
the suburbs feared they might be drawn into a formal arrangement that
would expose them to the city's problems. This fear was apparently greater
than their aversion to any but the lowest cost. According to a study by the
commissioner of health of Metropolis, a system of ambulance and paramedic teams serving on a countywide basis would most efficiently and effectively serve all the residents. These units would operate without regard

for municipal boundaries. The suburbs, however, preferred a plan based on the World War II civil defense zones used by the County Emergency Government Office's disaster plan, which gave the separate municipalities responsibility for directing the services that affected them. Though the "zone concept" required municipalities to cooperate within zones, it also isolated the city as a separate zone. It enabled the suburbs to share in the county plan without becoming entangled with the city. Opponents of the zone concept argued that it would create an inefficient distribution of work loads (crews in some zones would make too few runs to keep their skills sharp), require somewhat longer response times, and be more costly to operate. Nevertheless, the zone concept was adopted.

The adoption of the zone concept was to some extent due to the make-up of the council. The majority of the council members were suburban residents, even though the majority of the council's constituents were not. Nearly two-thirds (64 percent) of the county's million residents lived in the city.[2] However, only seven (41 percent) of seventeen council members at the start (two seats were vacant and two members did not give home addresses) were city residents. The geographic disproportion occurred because the members of the council were appointed to represent not only municipal governments but also health care and other organizations; many of these organizational leaders were suburban residents. Thus, for example, the physician who represented the Medical Society was also sympathetic to the interests of Riverview, the suburb in which he lived, although his support of the suburban perspective was not formally recognized.

The zone concept decentralized the EMS system and at the same time restricted the opportunities of ambulance workers. A countywide EMS corps, because of its size alone, might have established uniform patterns of recruitment and advancement that would have made the work a plausible career for an interested person. The geographically fragmented operation that the council chose, however, offered neither ready access nor multiple achievement levels.

Finances were a major concern of the council, because inflation and rising unemployment had begun to diminish tax revenues. Though a few citizens' groups spoke out for a paramedic system, they did not want higher taxes; the mayor of Metropolis vetoed the proposed paramedic program because of its cost but was overruled by the city's Common Council. The municipalities were eager to have the county take on the tax burden of raising the money for the program, though they did not want to relinquish any of their local control. Specific proposals ranged from those in which the county would bear 100 percent of the cost to those in which the municipalities would bear at least 50 percent. The final compromise had the county underwriting 75 percent of the costs (for training, salaries, maintenance, and communications), while the local governments paid the other 25 percent (for emergency vehicles and fringe benefits of personnel).

Financial considerations not only got a great deal of explicit attention in discussions, they also implicitly determined the direction of the council's efforts. The council concentrated on projects that could be financed from outside sources. For example, one of its first actions was to promote an EMS communications system in which the state would pay for the hardware. Federal moneys were available to the College of Medicine and to County Hospital for the training of paramedics, so the paramedics were treated as distinct from the basic EMTs. The medical community and the public seemed to find the paramedics more interesting than the basic EMTs. Equivalent effort was not put into a 911 emergency dispatch system, for example, or into a countywide system of basic EMTs. This concentration on paramedics was significant for the ambulance workers, because it allowed the two levels of EMS (basic and advanced) to develop somewhat independently and essentially eliminated a routine ladder of promotion between them. (In Metropolis the basic EMTs respond to most calls first and the paramedics respond only if the case is judged life-threatening.)

Finances were important again in the council's decisions about who should have *control over the field operations* of the system. The members wanted to minimize the start-up costs, as well as to get underway as soon as possible and to insure close medical supervision of the personnel. This last consideration seemed to keep them from seriously thinking about subsidizing private ambulance companies to provide EMS services, though many of the members were probably otherwise strong advocates of private enterprise. The reasoning seemed to be that a public agency would allow authorities closer control over the quality of services than would a private provider. A suggestion that the city's department of health might oversee EMS operations was dismissed without much discussion. A program under that department would have to start from scratch, since it had no resources in the field; such an approach would take too long (thus risking the loss of state and federal grants available at the moment) and would cost too much. The other public services—police and firefighters—were already involved in ambulance work in one place or another. The fire departments in particular had suitable garages and vehicles in most sectors. While the municipalities could presumably designate whatever agency they wanted to handle EMS, the trend was clearly toward fire departments. The only established paramedics in the county worked with the fire departments in the suburbs of Riverview and Clymer. (Dr. Kardijan maintained that the National Association of Fire Chiefs was a potent force in moving things in this direction.) The movement locally had its clearest expression when in 1977 the Common Council of Metropolis voted to abolish the police ambulance service and to vest authority for EMS in the fire department. (The County Council, which had been asked for advice, was careful to stay clear of the city's decision.) The resolution included private ambulance companies in the system to transport non-life-threatening cases to the hospital.

The council's decisions satisfied the political needs of the moment but did not necessarily establish the most effective or efficient EMS system. Perhaps the persons least well served were the ambulance workers. For Liberty attendants and for all other EMTs in the county, these decisions meant that careers in the prehospital phase of emergency medicine ceased to exist. Private companies were kept on the margin and limited to the basic EMT role. Anyone who wanted to go further would have to do so within a fire department, even though the paramedics received little support from their fellow firefighters.

Thus costs were controlled in the short run by piggybacking EMS operations on resources already in place rather than creating an independent and unique service. In most cases this meant that EMS work would be a secondary concern of organizations that considered their primary mission fire suppression. It also meant the EMS work would be further fragmented—divided not only by political boundaries and by distinct basic and advanced programs, but also among different organizations (fire departments, private ambulance companies, and hospital emergency departments).

Structural Lag

The fragmentation resulting from these divisions seems to be one cause of the disjunctions in service described in Chapter 7. It is probably typical of EMS systems in the United States. Most can be described as suffering from *structural lag*—the resources for achieving widely accepted goals are available but are not effectively employed, because existing social structures resist the modifications necessary to coordinate their use.[3] The term refers to the social paralysis that occurs when groups share an ideal or goal but not organizational interests. It is similar to William F. Ogburn's concept of "cultural lag": "A cultural lag occurs when one of two parts of culture which are correlated changes before or in greater degree than the other part does, thereby causing less adjustment between the two parts than existed previously."[4] However, where Ogburn's concept emphasizes differential rates of change, structural lag stresses resistance to recognized and desired change.

The 911 emergency phone system is an example of structural lag in Metropolis. No one denies that a universally recognized, three-digit number would be easier for the public to remember than the unexceptional seven-digit numbers of the police and fire departments. Certainly visitors unfamiliar with local conditions would be better served. The current system in Metropolitan County does not offer much support for a desperate caller in an emergency. A call from a pay phone (no coin required to dial 911) brought the following response:

So sorry. Your call cannot be completed as dialed. Please check the number and dial again, or call your operator to help you. This is a recording.

A call from a residential phone on another occasion was only slightly more expeditious:

(Dial 911. Sound of distant phone ringing once, twice, three times. Pause with no sound for nearly a minute. Then a woman's voice.)
Nine-One-One Emergency.
Hello? (Three more rings of the distant phone.)
Nine-One-One-Emergency.
Hello?
Do you want the police or the fire department?

Not only would a single emergency number avoid much of the confusion and speed the public's response, it would also allow for the training of special dispatchers. In pursuit of such advantages, the state passed a law mandating that all localities develop 911 systems by the end of 1987, and the East Central Health Systems Agency included specific objectives related to the systems in its 1981–82 Annual Implementation Plan (AIP).[5]

Along with general support for a 911 system, there was also specific resistance. The resisters did not deny the likely benefits of a single number, rather they emphasized the disadvantages. Neither the fire department nor the police department wanted to give up any control over dispatching functions. And the separate municipal governments were again fearful that the required cooperation would compromise their autonomy. They could accept the idea, but the social structures to which they were committed constrained them from implementing it.[6]

In the first years of the County Council's EMS plan the consequences of structural lag became evident. In many respects the system was working. The paramedic program, for example, was said to have successfully resuscitated a greater proportion of pulseless nonbreathers than the more celebrated programs in Seattle and Miami.[7] The first response combination of rescue squads and private ambulances had significantly cut the number of unnecessary runs in the city. At the same time, critical observers (especially the private attendants) saw problems with the program. It was not that anyone could prove that an alternative plan would be without shortcomings, and they admitted that the present system was saving lives, but they argued that an improved system would save more lives.

Three examples of structural lag in the fire department come up repeatedly in the conversations of the Liberty attendants—the marginal position of EMS in the department, the disinterest of firefighters in EMS, and the inability of interested people to become paramedics. The *marginality* of EMS is demonstrated in several ways. First, although the department makes more runs for medical emergencies than for fire suppression (on an "average" day in Metropolis in 1978 there were 78 fire calls, of which 40 were false alarms, and there were 82 rescue squad runs),[8] no senior official is solely in charge of EMS. Second, medical services are not part of the department's primary mission. When asked how the department would respond to a 20 percent across-the-board cut in the city budget, the fire chief said he would have to eliminate the (EMS) squads as well as some firefighting companies. "A budget reduction of this type, with the greatly reduced fire protection, would naturally result in a much higher property loss and the potential for an increased loss of life with the complete elimination of rescue squad service for the people of the community."[9] A discussion in quarters a month earlier had accurately anticipated the fire chief's comments.

Someone said Liberty should be supporting efforts to put a limit on taxes. If it means cuts in service, the "frills" would go first, the "extras." And EMS would probably be one of these. The fire department would cut out their EMT programs. That in turn would mean the privates would get the runs, and Liberty would benefit! Example of tunnel vision or worldly wisdom?

This view received some support six months later; when the firefighters threatened to go on strike, everyone on the Liberty roster was put on alert, because the privates were expected to handle the total EMS load, including first response. Third, the department does not give much weight to EMT status. Transfers within the department often ignore emergency medical skills. A firefighter reported that during one major shift, seniority rather than other qualifications determined who should be assigned to the "Crash Fire Rescue" unit at Metropolitan International Airport, with the result that EMTs were replaced by untrained personnel.

Structural lag is also obvious in the failure of the fire department to alter its career lines to accommodate its responsibility for EMS. As a result, firefighters are not eager to undertake the work. They get little or no *recognition* for their extra training and heavier work loads.

Joe had worked with the fire department in Riverview. They had required EMT training so he had taken the course earlier and was being reexamined. He has been with the Metropolis Fire Department for just a year. After he gets his patch [passes the National Registry exam] he'll probably go on the rescue squads, though he doesn't want to. What he doesn't like about the squads is that they have to run all night. An engine company might get one call but a squad gets a lot. He says the rescue squads aren't all that popular among the firefighters, though some guys do like rescue work.

The EMT-firefighters are not given extra pay, nor can they stay with emergency work and still be promoted. The local of the International Association of Firefighters does not support the paramedics' attempts to receive higher pay than nonparamedics. The results can be seen in the attrition rate: of the fifty-two firefighters trained as paramedics, twenty-two (42 percent) quit within the first three years of the program, leaving the service 18 persons short.[10] The paramedics complain that they need leadership within the department and on each unit, promotion opportunities within the program, support to prevent "burnout," and that they deserve premium pay. The firefighters' union president is not sympathetic: "A lot of them think they are entitled to more money. But they fail to realize they are firefighters first. Nobody is forcing anybody to be a paramedic. They don't have to worry about a roof falling in or a floor dropping out or the smoke and the fire." To which a former paramedic responded: "A firefighter's job is physical. A paramedic has a high-stress, mental job. You are making a lot more medical decisions than you realize."[11]

As the Liberty attendants see it, not only are people within the MFD carrying out EMS functions reluctantly, people who would like to do the work are prevented by institutional *barriers*. The most obvious barrier is the requirement that a person must be a firefighter before being a paramedic. The people most clearly disadvantaged by the requirement are females. The Metropolis Fire Department has no female firefighters. Recognizing at least this aspect of the problem, a federal judge in December of 1979 ordered the city to allow women to apply for paramedic jobs without first passing training courses required for firefighters. Helen Laber had been working on the cars with Liberty for about a year when she took the test for the paramedics.

I passed everything except the physical strength part. I couldn't lift the weight they required. I don't know what it was; for some reason I was tired that day and wasn't performing well. But it was much more than one would ever have to lift in the course of the work. And I didn't really want to move into the city anyway. We're settled in Fairhaven now and after fourteen years of moving around I'd just as soon stay where we are.

As a result of the court ruling, some women have been admitted to para-medic training, though all the problems of structural lag have not thereby been resolved.

In the opinion of the Liberty attendants, the EMS system has been snarled in an organizational tangle that defeats their aspirations and fails to provide the best care. They are frustrated because they cannot advance within the line of work they like, and because the firefighters seem to dis-like having that work forced upon them. The crews figure that since every-one seems to be frustrated, the quality of care cannot be as good as it might be.

Regulation

The politics of EMS did not stop with the County Council's creation of a new system. The county passed along the responsibility for implementing and supervising the system to the city and state, which exercised their duties through the routine politics of regulatory agencies.

For the most part, the effects of routine political maneuvering reach the attendants only indirectly through their employers. The crews are wit-nesses rather than participants in what occurs. They are directly contacted by state or national agencies about their individual professional status and not much else. This occurs, for example, when they receive a letter of con-gratulations for having passed the Registry's written examination, or an "Envo-gram" warning them that they must produce evidence of having met continuing education requirements by December 31st, or a rubber-stamped form notifying them that they are no longer included on the roster of a provider and therefore cannot have their state license renewed. The attendants are aware of other political decisions that affect their work life only if they make an effort to find out about them or hear about them indi-rectly through the grapevine or the media. Yet decisions in these realms can cause the company to alter its work load, reduce the number of employees, or even go out of business.

The city agency with the most influence over the fate of Liberty atten-dants is the Utilities and Licenses Committee, which makes recommenda-tions for action to the Common Council. It is this committee that sets the private EMS companies' fees; these largely determine the privates' profit margin, which in turn affects the wages and benefits of the privates' employees.

After two years of operation, the privates asked for a $10.00 increase in the flat rate they charged for EMS service within the county. Six months later, they requested permission to charge patients for expendable medical supplies (bandages, splints, oxygen), for mileage to a hospital more than three-and-one-half miles from the scene, and for emergency runs in which no conveyance is necessary. Within the next six months, they asked for another increase in the flat rate. Harold from Liberty, who was joined by the other owners after he made the original request, presented the case this way:

The simple fact is that the [$75] fee that was set in January '78 when the system got underway was lower than we were used to charging. I'll be honest with you. It was profitable during '78. And it was marginally profitable during '79. But since September [1979] I've lost $15,000 per quarter—a cash operating loss.[12]

Part of the financial difficulty of the privates stems from their inability to collect from all the patients they carry. Some of the patients refuse to pay because the ambulance was summoned by the firefighters and the patients assumed there would be no charge. Although the privates collect on 85 percent of their routine transfers, unpaid bills for emergency calls vary from 37 percent to 66 percent for the four companies. In 1978 Liberty failed to collect on 41 percent of its emergency runs.[13]

The Common Council has never been eager to raise ambulance rates. Members are uneasy about whether the charges are justified, about whether the patients will get insurance coverage, about public reaction. Although the council has the authority to deny an increase, however, it is not unambiguously in a position of strength. The city needs the private companies. If the privates dropped out of the EMS system, the city would have to buy, house, and maintain 18 additional ambulances and staff them with 144 EMTs (8 persons per ambulance for round-the-clock coverage), at a start-up cost estimated by the commissioner of health to be about $4 million. When the council attempted to postpone a decision on the most recent increase request, Harold gently threatened:

I don't want to put them under the gun. Suffice it to say that I'm operating in the red and I can't do it anymore. I have to have a profit. We should not be making an obscene profit. But we should be making a profit. I don't care how they [the Common Council] do it, as long as the bottom line is black.[14]

As costs have risen with inflation, the companies have moved into a cycle in which they receive permission for an increase and immediately initiate a request for another. The requests are reminders of the city's authority over the privates; the permissions, of its dependence on them. The relationship, which appears stable on the surface for the moment, may in fact be shaky.

The regulatory powers of the city are also displayed when complaints about the ambulance service receive public attention. It has become routine for the privates in the field to make most of the emergency conveyances, while the rescue squads make almost none. The few mobile (paramedic) units are too busy to make conveyances unless absolutely necessary. However, this practice was evidently neither noticed nor understood by the politicians until they were forced to look at it.[15] In one case the newspaper reported that a private crew had carried a critical patient who had later died. A follow-up on this story led to the discovery that the four private companies participating in the EMS system had never been officially certified, as required by the new city ordinances. The council put some pressure on the commissioner of health, who quickly negotiated a certification of the companies in connection with a compromise on rates.

In a later case a distant relative of one of the city aldermen died two-and-one-half hours after arriving at the hospital. The alderman contended that the man might not have died if he had been treated by paramedics on the scene rather than handled by a private ambulance crew. Though the fire department said the rescue squad EMTs who examined the patient found him stable and in no imminent danger of death, the alderman was angry:

This incident very definitely points up a very serious problem with the first and second response of the emergency medical system within the city of Metropolis. It seems to me that the Fire Department has repeatedly opted to use private ambulances in lieu of their rescue squads for reasons which are very unclear to me. It would seem to me that conveyance should be made [by the fire department] in all potential life-threatening situations; and if the city of Metropolis does not have the ability to handle that volume of calls, additional rescue squads should be added so as to maintain the integrity of a total EMS system.[16]

The council took no action in this latter case beyond calling for an investigation by the commissioner of health. There was no serious political infighting. However, the few statements that were made demonstrated to the crews that the council did not understand how the EMS system was operating. In particular, neither politicians nor the public recognized that the rescue squads and the private ambulances offered the same level of training (basic EMT). A clear implication of the statements was that the privates were under suspicion of being incompetent.

The Liberty crews' morale, work assignments, incomes, and futures are all affected by city politics. First, suggestions that the private companies might be cheating the public, and the implication that the skills of the attendants are deficient, bother them. Second, the paperwork has changed as the city and the companies have worked out different arrangements. The attendants might or might not have to add the cost of expendable supplies, calculate a surcharge for extra mileage, or assess a fee for a "no transport." Third, the attendants' requests for raises or benefits are countered by the companies' claims of financial difficulty, which depend in part on the city's regulation of fees. Finally, the struggles with the city continually remind the crews of the precariousness of their jobs.

The State Division of Health is also a powerful force in the work life of the attendant, but it is more distant and seems more predictable than the city agencies. In most cases the state simply implements regulations required by the federal government as a condition of certain grants. An example is KKK-A-1822, the federal specification for ambulances, which includes such details as the broad orange band required for identification.[17] In enforcing these regulations, the state sometimes draws the criticism of locals, as when a relatively new ambulance serving one of the Metropolitan suburbs was not approved because its roof was three-and-one-half inches lower than the required fifty-two inches. The Liberty crews consider some of the state regulations to be bureaucratic busywork; the ambulance inspections, for example, are nearly a joke.

Jardine said Liberty's ambulances were inspected by the state last month. He said the inspectors were concerned about whether we had three-inch tape, about whether there were safety pins in the trauma boxes, and about the length of the padded board splints. The state wouldn't want them to be a quarter-inch too long, he said. On the other hand, a shoulder harness for the crew seats is not required even though, according to Jardine, the chances of an accident go up 300 to 500 percent when the red lights and siren are turned on. [Liberty's cars passed the inspection.]

The ultimate source of other regulations is unclear, but the crews assign the blame to the state. B.Z. told some of us:

It is no longer recommended [by authorities on emergency medicine] to use a foot-and-ankle splint at all. They do not sufficiently immobilize the movement of the foot. We should use at least a half-leg splint. We carry the foot-and-ankle only because the state requires it.

The state claims that lack of money prevents it from carrying out its functions properly. An example is the inability of the Department of EMS Systems to maintain an up-to-date assessment of the ambulance services in the state by processing the EMT reports routinely sent to it. Thus the state is forced to ignore a potentially valuable means of quality control.

The state's Department of EMS Systems requires that new people qualify as EMTs according to National Registry standards, but once qualified they can renew their state licenses without meeting certification requirements simply by remaining on the roll of a provider and reapplying each year. This position might have been due to a concern that stricter recertification requirements would diminish the number of available EMTs, particularly among volunteers. This concern was also evident in a 1979 attempt to pass legislation that would allow relatively untrained people to staff ambulances in communities of less than 10,000 population. The effort was opposed by the State Emergency Medical Technicians' Association, which appealed to its members to contact their legislators on the matter.[18]

The crews comply with the state regulations that are unavoidable and joke about those they consider silly. Overall, they seem to consider the state less demanding than either city or national agencies.

Professional Politics

Two kinds of professional politics that touch the attendants' lives are more distant from them than either the city or the state: the activities of career politicians with an interest in EMS and EMS professionals with an interest in politics. The former create federal legislation and establish and disestablish federal agencies with authority over the nation's EMS workers. The latter engage in struggles for the right to define the state of the art within EMS.

There is no denying the potency of the federal government in shaping EMS. Douglas's well-informed study of ambulance work in the late 1960s gives no hint of the swift and profound changes that would take place in the following decade under the pressure of federal regulations, grants, and threats of funding cuts.[19] Indeed, the Liberty attendants occupy a formal status (EMT) that would not have existed except for this pressure. The federal influence has been noted throughout this account—on the availability of emergency services, on standards of training, on specifications for ambulances.

Federal policies, however, are as unstable as they are potent. A top priority of one administration or one congress may be considered expendable by a successor. Such was the experience of EMS. It received strong support from Washington during the 1970s but, with the faltering of the economy and the shifting of political power at the end of that period, it lost its advocates. (The Liberty workers at the time of this study had benefited more from the period of support than they had suffered from the period of retrenchment.) President Reagan's stringent budget policies have most seriously reduced federal support. There is an irony in the fact that the president benefited directly from the capital's EMS system when he was treated for gunshot wounds following the attempt on his life in the spring of 1981.[20] Moreover, during a campaign tour in Milwaukee in 1980, Reagan saw a listener collapse during a streetcorner speech. The president-to-be asked if there were a doctor present and, having been told someone had called the paramedics, then asked for a moment of silent prayer. When the paramedics signaled that the man was all right, and before he resumed his speech, Reagan said, "This is the kind of service the government should be supporting."[21] Presumably he was referring to local rather than to federal government.

The diminishing of interest in EMS can be seen on several fronts. The Department of Health and Human Services faces reduced support generally. Within that department, the Division of EMS, which oversaw granting programs, was transformed into the Program Office for EMS and placed under the administration of the Bureau of Community Health, an agency somewhat out of favor with the new conservatives. The Interagency Committee on EMS, established to coordinate the many EMS-related programs scattered in many federal agencies, has gradually become inactive. EMS systems funding, which advocates feel is essential for providing direction to local areas, has been slated to be merged with other funds in block grants to the states, which would not be accountable for specific uses of the moneys. These developments are regarded as sufficiently ominous by professionals that over thirty EMS-related organizations have formed the EMS Coalition primarily for the purpose of lobbying in Washington, D.C.[22]

The effects of these federal policy shifts on local workers are delayed and indirect. Perhaps for this reason, the Liberty attendants are neither aware of nor interested in changes on the national scene. They do not talk, for example, about the possible consequences of the earlier reductions in EMS development grants. Many of the threatened federal programs deal with the cooperation of regional providers and the coordination of field operations, and thus concern administrative organization and communications. The Liberty attendants, who are part of an operating system, probably would not become aware of such changes until local tax increases and budget cuts emerged as obvious consequences. Reductions in other federal programs, such as Medicaid (which pays for many ambulance runs), could eventually affect the company's, and therefore its employees', income, but the crews do not seem to be worried. Their general view, apparently based on the immediate past, is an optimistic one that EMS will continue to expand and improve.

Political struggles within the profession also influence the EMTs' work. The struggles are of several kinds. Some involve only EMS organizations. An example of this type is the attempt of the National Registry to become the sole certification agency for EMTs. States that decide to promote their own certification examinations or that form certain kinds of reciprocity agreements are acting in opposition to the National Registry's aim. This political contest will ultimately determine the standards for qualifying as an EMT.

Other struggles are between providers of EMS knowledge (educators and researchers) or providers of EMS care (hospitals and prehospital operatives). Occasionally the former argue about the effectiveness of particular treatments. A prominent case is the dispute over the proper emergency treatment of the so-called "cafe coronary," choking on food (or some other obstruction in the airway). Dr. Henry J. Heimlich, a director of surgery and professor of advanced clinical sciences in Cincinnati, developed a modified bear-hug technique, which he claimed to be highly effective in dislodging obstructions in the throat. While suppliers have produced instructional posters and wallet cards on the technique, and while some states and some restaurant associations have trained their employees in it, the American Red Cross continues to promote the back-slap (or back blows) technique. Heimlich claims there is no evidence that back slaps are effective and some evidence they are harmful. In fact, he maintains that in this context "a back blow is a death blow." The Red Cross bases its position on recommendations of the National Academy of Science—National Research Council, and is supported by the American Heart Association and the American Medical Association.

The EMS worker could hardly escape the controversy. The Heimlich maneuver came to public attention in 1974 in time to be included in the second edition of the EMT text, *Emergency Care and Transportation of the Sick and Injured.*[23] The text presented it as an adjunct to back slaps, which was essentially an endorsement of the Red Cross position. At the same time, other material read by EMS workers gives considerable space to Heimlich's arguments, along with some criticisms of his evidence.[24] The inconclusiveness of the debate has left EMS instructors in the awkward situation of sometimes having to teach a procedure (the official text's recommendation of back slaps) that they feel is inferior to an alternative (the Heimlich maneuver).[25] Though ambulance attendants are not often called upon to treat choking victims, a responsibility usually forced on bystanders, they do trade opinions in quarters about the merits of the two sides.

Political struggles between providers of care can concern authority relations or responsibility for particular aspects of the work or the right to employ certain devices or techniques. While most of these contests are between physicians and paramedics or between hospitals and fire departments, the basic EMTs may be directly involved. Medical personnel question, for example, whether EMTs should be permitted to employ the MAST device at their own discretion. The physicians argue that the EMTs are not routinely trained to use MAST, that many emergency departments are not familiar with it, and that its effect on certain traumatic conditions can be anticipated only by physicians. Ambulance crews that have been carrying and using the MAST devices claim MAST has saved lives that would otherwise have been lost. The Liberty crews are familiarized with the MAST garment in in-service training. However, there are legal questions about whether the devices are within the ambulance attendant's established "scope of practice" or competence, and the interpretation of "scope of practice" varies with the local medical community.[26] Liberty ambulances continue to carry the devices, but the crews are cautioned against using them except in a critical situation.

These diverse political currents are continually shifting the ambulance attendants' situation. Yet the Liberty attendants make little effort to influence the currents. They seem to be aware of political actions that have a direct, immediate effect on their work, but they are not interested in political issues that have an indirect or long-range effect. The obvious channels of political expression for the crews are the state and national EMT associations. However, the Liberty attendants are reluctant to pay the dues and skeptical about what the associations can do for them. Consequently, while some of them attend training seminars, none of them ever talk about attending a meeting of an EMT organization. There are EMTs who are more active politically than those at Liberty, but evidently not many. The editors of the state *EMTA Journal* attempt in each issue to answer the question, "Why should we join the EMTA?" And as often as not they plaintively ask, "Is there anyone out there?"

Around Metropolis many of the EMTs are firefighters or police, whose concerns about job security, benefits, and career advancement are handled through their unions, or volunteers who pursue these concerns elsewhere. Thus, they do not help to make the EMT associations strong forces with regard to such matters. Moreover, some of them do not identify themselves as EMTs sufficiently to support even a "professional" interest in the associations. This division within the ranks of the EMTs hinders the development of a potent occupation-based movement. Perhaps as a result, the Liberty attendants are passive observers of the politics of EMS.

conclusion

Some Policy Implications

Just before you come into Mercer,
someone had scribbled a crude sign
that said: "Take it easy, driver—this
town has no hospital."
—Armand Cirilli, *Iron County Miner*

A case study of one company is not an adequate basis for making recommendations for public policy about ambulances. The single case is certainly not typical of all ambulance companies. It is not even typical of all private ambulance companies. In fact, in some important respects Liberty Ambulance Company is not like the other private companies in the same city. Moreover, the qualitative materials on which the description in this book is based are not amenable to the kinds of verification that can be used to "prove" points. Having acknowledged these limitations, I intend nevertheless to conclude by making some generalizations about ambulance work that have implications for public policy. I can justify these generalizations to my own satisfaction on two grounds. First, with all the variation from one work setting to another, there are still unavoidable similarities in ambulance work wherever it is found. Public expectations, financial resources, equipment design, training, and medical supervision exert constraints on what work can be done and on how it can be done. Therefore, with a modest knowledge of other companies and of the EMS literature, one should be able to discern in the details of one case those features that are common to ambulance work generally. Second, such generalizations as these need not be definitive in order to be useful. They can suggest improvements in EMS. And quite apart from their practical value, they can point to interesting subjects for speculation, debate, and investigation.

The Value of EMS

The evidence is clear that emergency medical care saves lives. We have both dramatic instances and carefully compiled statistics to back up the claim. A sampling of the headlines of paramedic rescue stories illustrates the former:

3 Life Stories: Why More Survive "Sudden Death"
Drowned Child Brought Back to Life
"Miracle Recovery" for Woman Frozen Solid
He Fought Back from the Shadow of Death
Under Water 50 Minutes, Boy, 8, Alive

The paramedic rate of "saves" of pulseless nonbreathers (Chapter 8) illustrates the latter. But these facts do not touch on two important questions about the values implied in EMS systems: Do we want to save the lives the ambulance workers rescue? Does the benefit of saving lives through EMS outweigh the cost?

The first question is raised dramatically by the story of Jardine's refusing to begin CPR on a dying patient (Chapter 6). It embodies the dilemma in

which, at the extremes, we are forced either to sustain all life indiscrimi-
nately or to choose arbitrarily to allow some but not others to die. Jardine's
case is exceptional, because the EMS system normally follows the former
option. The problem with this option is that we make it very difficult for
people to achieve death. Those who by any natural definition have
reached the end of their lives are kept alive sometimes for long periods
because it is more awkward routinely to discontinue life support measures
than it is routinely to initiate them.

One of the consequences of EMS is thus to prevent the earlier death of
people who will soon succumb anyway. Among the people who are kept
alive are many who are very elderly, very ill, or hopelessly damaged. We
can see this pattern in the record of Metropolitan County paramedics from
1973 to 1978 and their treatment of "sudden death," heart attacks that are
fatal in twenty-four hours or less.[1] The outcomes of a total of 1,100 cases
treated over that period were as follows:

500 were dead and unrevivable at the scene (46%)
350 were in ventricular fibrillation but could not be revived (32%)
135 had a semblance of normal heartbeat restored for short time (12%)
57 survived with slight or massive brain damage (5%)
58 survived without impairment (5%)

These figures show that half of the "salvaged" patients suffered slight or
massive brain damage. The system is not simply rescuing threatened individuals; it is at the same time rescuing ailing and dependent individuals.
This reality is somewhat at odds with the popular image of ambulance services saving vigorous and blameless individuals from dire circumstances.
Among Metropolitan County ambulance patients, as many are victims of
the failures of their own bodies (heart attacks, strokes, diabetes) as are victims of accidental injury. And many of the younger patients, those who
engage in high-risk behaviors, such as drug abuse, driving while drinking,
and mishandling firearms, are victims of their own stupidity rather than of
random misfortune.

From this skeptical outlook, one can view the complete elimination of
EMS as a way of allowing the forces of accident, disaster, and infirmity to
thin the population. This radical step, in keeping with the epigraph at the
beginning of the chapter, would emphasize individual responsibility. It
would have the effect of reducing that proportion of the society that survives in a state of unpromising dependence on medical support. It would
also allow an increase in the tragedies of untimely death.

Between the extremes of allowing EMS to run out of control or eliminat-
ing it is the possibility of establishing standards for judging when to apply
life-saving techniques. Appropriate standards would allow some lives to

end while requiring a supreme effort to sustain others. The informal standards that presently guide behavior (for example, in determining when to discontinue CPR) are not explicitly acknowledged, carefully developed, or uniformly employed. The problems of developing such standards have already been faced in the patient selection procedures for scarce life-saving techniques, such as renal dialysis.[2] The problems have not all been solved, but reasonable solutions are within reach. Some such standards are necessary if EMS is going to help raise the health status of the society rather than simply salvage warm bodies.

Standards for deciding who shall be saved are essential, because we do not have sufficient resources to save everyone. This observation brings us to the second value question we posed: Are the benefits of EMS worth the costs? The romantic reply is that if we can save even one life by our efforts, then it is worth it. Unfortunately, because our resources are limited, the effort we put into one project is potentially lost to another. The funds we invest in an open-heart surgery unit will undoubtedly save lives, but the funds are no longer available for a prenatal care program, which could have saved other lives. Are the funds invested in EMS well spent, or would they be of greater benefit elsewhere?

The direct costs of EMS are not great compared with other forms of medical care. Some argue that support of EMS would have a greater payoff in lives saved than nearly any other medical investment.[3] Even a report by General Motors (apparently arguing against the cost-effectiveness of government regulations on automobiles) claimed that a quality ambulance system would be the least expensive of more than sixty life-extending programs studied.[4] The direct costs of EMS may appear to be substantial when a community considers adding start-up costs and maintenance to the programs it is already funding. But in comparison with other medical operations, ambulance services can be seen to be more economical.

The complaints of the Liberty attendants about shit calls suggest one way in which the cost of ambulance service can be pushed up. Abuse of the system may force either an increase in resources or a curtailment of services. As 911 telephone systems have produced more traffic, police departments have stopped using patrol cars to respond to every call.[5] There are even jokes about installing coin-operated fire alarms. Two other items that could reasonably be associated with EMS would indirectly enlarge its costs. One is the hospital component with its trained staff and sophisticated technology, the emergency departments and intensive care units, without which the ambulance services would be less effective. The second item is the cost of caring for badly damaged victims who survive because of EMS but who have no prospect of regaining their human capacities. When these indirect costs are taken into account, EMS might not seem such an economically attractive package, though it is probably still a better buy than most other medical treatments.

The benefits of ambulance services are not restricted to saving lives, although that aspect of the work gets the most public (and professional) attention. Ambulance attendants provide an enormously important service in their efforts to limit physical damage. Using proper techniques to stabilize injuries and move patients can prevent further harm and possibly avoid permanent disability (for example, paralysis of the legs if a back injury is not handled properly). The magnitude of these preventive benefits is difficult to document, but we should not ignore them. The contributions of the basic EMTs, like those employed by Liberty, are largely of this kind. It would be a serious error to emphasize the treatment of problems that are immediately life-threatening to the extent that we ignore the threat to the quality of future life by less obvious problems.

Finally, we need to recognize that EMS has a value for society that is not strictly medical. Ambulance service is also a symbol of the community's regard for human life. Ambulance work provides an opportunity for people to serve the community, and ambulance workers, particularly volunteers but also those employees who are willing to work for low wages, are themselves an indicator of social solidarity within the community.[6] In addition to its practical applications, then, EMS may well be a booster of the public morale, a benefit not necessarily less real or important than products that are more easily quantified.

The Organization of Care

If we are going to have an EMS system, we should realize that some forms of organization will be more efficient than others. The Liberty case shows at least two ways in which social arrangements interfere with effective ambulance work. The first concerns the auspices under which the prehospital phase of service is carried out, and the second concerns the coordination of the several organizational components of the system.

Liberty Ambulance Company cannot offer its employees any hope for future advancement, therefore they are forced to write off their training and accomplishments and look for work elsewhere. The EMTs in the fire department are in a somewhat similar situation. For the firefighters, EMS is not a route to promotion, even if they are trained as paramedics. Indeed, EMS work is at best a detour, and perhaps even a barrier, on the road to advancement. At the very worst, it is perceived as a punishment by those who are forced into the work because the department does not have enough volunteers. The situation is deplorable, because the way ambulance services are organized keeps everyone's morale unnecessarily low.

The root of the problem in Metropolis seems to be that EMS is an add-on. The primary responsibility for the local services was added on to the fire department, and the private companies were added on to back up the department. None of those who work in the field are able to feel they are performing a service that is recognized as valuable and worthy of support. The fire department claims to have adopted EMS enthusiastically, but its recruitment, training, promotions, leadership, and self-image (some EMTs ride the rescue squads in firefighter's gear) are all oriented to fire suppression. Liberty is running a backup operation with employees who are trained for, and who aspire to, first-responder status. None of those who work in the field are able to see the value of the work they are doing reflected in support from their own organization. The individual EMT's idealism and that of his fellow workers provides much of the incentive to continue.

In addition to depressing morale, the lack of organizational support encourages high turnover among the EMTs. In the fire department they leave the rescue squads and the mobile units to rejoin engine and ladder companies. At Liberty they quit and find other jobs. Turnover not only raises questions in the minds of new recruits, it also deprives them of experienced colleagues who could serve as teachers and role models. The possibility of increasing ambulance worker competence through the sharing of knowledge on the job is diminished where the turnover of personnel is high, and ultimately the quality of patient care suffers.

If this line of reasoning is correct, then it is important to organize ambulance services in such a way that the personnel can believe in the integrity and value of the work (that it is not secondary) and have some prospect that the effort they invest in gaining competence will be rewarded (that there can be career advancement). The payoff will be in higher worker morale and better quality of care.

Ambulance work is affected not only by the structure of sponsoring organizations, but also by how the participating organizations mesh. The Liberty crews are part of a system that includes two training programs, a dozen hospitals, the fire department, and four private ambulance companies, but no strong leadership. The fire department has the authority to coordinate the system, but not the inclination. Since each of the participating organizations has its own mission, knowledge, and techniques, it should not surprise us that cooperation among them requires some effort. Largely as a result of the lack of coordination, the Liberty crews experience, and contribute to, misunderstandings, delays, mistakes, and irresponsibility in carrying out EMS functions. The workers involved in these failures are neither malicious nor stupid; they are simply committed to the aims and routines of their own organizations rather than to some encompassing but abstract goal. Unfortunately such diverse commitments often lead to suspicion, competition, and antagonism.

Probably the ideal arrangement would be to have all the components of EMS included under a single organizational umbrella, so that a particular office would have both the responsibility and the authority to see that the activities of the separate units were coordinated. Given the existing health care institutions in most communities, it is unlikely that this ideal arrangement of new programs will often be realized. But at least the system should have a coordinator committed primarily to EMS rather than to one of its components. Moreover, the personnel from the different organizations should be required to share some of their training, continuing education, and in-service programs, and encouraged to observe and participate in other work settings. Regularly scheduled critique sessions involving all components would probably be helpful. Only occasionally does the Metropolis system include any of these cooperative ventures.

The number of abuse calls Liberty handles may indicate that the public is simply ignorant of the purpose of the emergency ambulance services. A strong coordinator could devise the means to keep an appropriate image of the EMS system in the minds of the populace. Part of the public education project could be aimed at the medical community, informing physicians of the capabilities of EMTs and paramedics. In a fragmented EMS operation no one is responsible for such projects. Without an agency that sees its mission as coordination, the coordination does not get done.

Quality Control

Liberty Ambulance Company does not have any routine measures for checking the quality of patient care, nor does the city, nor the state. My impression is that the fire department does not make quality control checks on the rescue squad EMTs either. (The work of the paramedics is evaluated more closely, because they are acting on authority delegated by physicians and because the physicians publish professional reports on the efficiency of the paramedics.) However, even without reliable evidence, the ambulance workers are suspect in the eyes of some people, and criticisms are not hard to find. Part of the problem is that the attendants are assessed according to different expectations by their peers, the police, their instructors, ED personnel, city officials, the public, firefighters, and the company owners. Because they are relatively low in professional status, ambulance workers are answerable to these incongruent expectations; if they were higher in status, they could establish their own definition of the nature of their work. A routine mechanism of quality control might well dissipate suspicions about the ambulance attendants and establish their area of competence. By doing so, it could contribute to the institutionalization of ambulance work and thus to the reduction of conflicting expectations.

While regular quality checks might improve patient care, it is questionable whether additional regulations based on such checks could be effective. First, it is impossible to draw up regulations that cover all circumstances, especially where the demands of the work are varying and unpredictable. Second, enforcement of such regulations is costly; Liberty is relatively free of outside evaluation, because responsible agencies claim they do not have resources for more careful scrutiny. Third, the crucial part of ambulance work is done in the field where, for all practical purposes, it is out of the reach of inspectors. Fourth, some important aspects of patient care—gentleness and emotional comfort, for example—are difficult to assess, even by close observation.

My experience at Liberty persuaded me that the quality of ambulance work could be enhanced by encouraging the idealism with which most of the workers arrive and by promoting the conditions that make good patient care possible. The Liberty attendants who are competent and effective also talk about their work with pride. With some encouragement from the ambulance worker's organization and his community, this kind of pride in work might be sustained rather than allowed to turn gradually into cynicism. Adequate pay and occasional compliments are both practical and symbolic indicators of the kind of support that makes work seem worthwhile.

Creating the conditions for good patient care would include maximizing the attendant's empathy for his patients. The sociocultural distance between attendant and patient often makes empathy difficult. Liberty's crews are mostly young, white, middle-class males, while a large proportion of their patients are elderly, nonwhite, poor, or working-class females. A significant number of Liberty patients speak Spanish, but none of the crews do. If recruitment, training, and employment were aimed at producing an EMT pool that more nearly represented the patient population of the service area, ambulance worker empathy and thus the quality of patient care might be improved. It would improve because of better understanding between those employees and clients who have similar characteristics and because the social heterogeneity within the crew culture would raise the consciousness of all the workers.

An important barrier to achieving a representative EMT corps is the exclusion of some categories of aspiring workers because of the irrelevant requirements of sponsoring organizations. In Metropolis one has to be skilled in fire suppression before one can be considered for paramedic training. Further, no female and few nonwhites have ever qualified as firefighters. An obvious consequence of this situation is to maintain a relatively homogeneous department quite unrepresentative of the service area. While this discrepancy might not affect the quality of fire suppression work, there is antecdotal evidence that it does affect the attitude of rescue squad members toward certain kinds of patients and thus perhaps the quality of care. Candidates for ambulance work should be screened fairly and solely on the basis of qualifications pertinent to the specific job. Standards of dexterity, strength, and intelligence that are much higher than the requirements of normal practice are obstacles that artificially exclude certain kinds of people.

Personnel

The quality of patient care is compromised by the high rate of turnover in ambulance work because much of the workers' skill is a result of on-the-job training and is lost when rookie EMTs take over. The problem is compounded when the replacements do not want to do ambulance work but are forced into it because there are not enough volunteers to fill the necessary slots, as is the case with the Metropolis Fire Department. The turnover problem at Liberty (and to a large extent in the fire department) is mainly a matter of pay and prospects. However, high attrition rates and short careers seem to be common among ambulance workers, even where promotion and benefits are reasonable. One explanation for this phenomenon rests on the assumption that ambulance work requires people who are idealistic, who are willing and eager to serve those in need by performing unpleasant tasks. People who will do the job properly are supposedly not attracted by pay alone; they do the work because they are dedicated. This dedication or commitment or idealism is sufficiently fragile that it weakens without support and is destroyed by the adverse conditions the workers must routinely face.[7] The more dedicated they are the more they suffer from the inevitable stress of high stakes and uncertain outcomes. Since the stressful conditions of the work are unlikely to change, the remedy for these complaints must be in altering the worker's expectations and backing. A more realistic preview during training of the nature of work on the streets and more encouragement from medical personnel, together with opportunities for emotional ventilation with coworkers on the job, might enable workers who are burning out to reestablish psychic equilibrium.

A related explanation for turnover is that too much training can lead to overqualified personnel who have lower job satisfaction and lower morale.[8] This seems an apt description of the Liberty EMTs, whose training emphasizes the importance of careful patient assessment and basic life support for first responders, but whose jobs require them to receive non-life-threatening cases from the fire department for transportation. Ambulance workers in this position may well be discouraged, because the distinctiveness of their job is diminished. They are left with a combination of duties no different (except in rewards) from those of other occupations; they drive like teamsters, lift and carry like stevedores, and prepare forms like clerks. They begin to suspect that they are simply doing someone else's dirty work, and they try to prop up their self-esteem by exaggerating their own accomplishments. Liberty EMTs occasionally have an opportunity to operate as first responders and handle patients in critical condition; these events seem to provide them with an incentive to endure the less interesting work. Their experience supports the idea that workers ought to have the opportunity to exercise the range of skills in which they have been trained. It suggests that a system in which EMTs are responsible for both first response and transportation may produce higher worker morale than a situation in which those tasks are discontinuous and where some crews are restricted to the less demanding work.

Implications for Sociology

This study was intended to be a detailed examination of the social conditions that shape ambulance work. At the same time it is reasonable to suppose that a sociological investigation of this sort can teach us not only about the subject under scrutiny but also about sociology. Since there is not now a body of sociological literature on ambulances or even on emergency medical services, the contributions of this study cannot be specific. But there are at least three ways in which this work adds to our general sociological knowledge.

First, the study provides data from a heretofore unexamined area of social activity in support of a variety of current sociological inferences. Central among these supportive findings (most of which are indicated in the text by footnote references) are the following. That social realities (medical emergencies) are largely constructed from the performances of the actors. That many consumers misuse public services (emergency medical services) to fulfill needs they cannot satisfy by other means. That providers of services (emergency medical technicians) are influenced by nonprofessional values (ethnic and class culture) in dealing with their clients. That the social dislocation of workers (EMTs) on irregular shifts has serious social (family life) and physical (jet lag) consequences for themselves and for their work (patient care). That barriers to promotion (EMTs) lead to career instability and high rates of turnover, which result in the loss of experienced (on-the-job) workers and thus lower quality work (patient care). That ineffective coordination of provider organizations (emergency medical service systems) is costly to a community in time, money, morale, and quality of services (patient care). That urban areas are at a disadvantage when suburban areas control supposedly neutral administrative bodies (county council on emergency medical services).

Second, the study indicates that some modifications in traditional sociological concepts might be useful. It shows that attributes that have been associated with professional occupations (ideal of service, autonomy in decision making) are present in some blue-collar work. Indeed, some blue-collar workers volunteer their time and energy, endure personal inconvenience, and even engage in deviant activities (the five-finger discount) to further their occupational missions. Such workers might be described accurately as *blue-collar professionals*. The findings of the study also suggest that a new category—*emergency service workers*—is called for in the study of work and occupations. This category, which comprises police, fire fighters, EMTs, ED personnel, search and rescue workers, disaster relief workers, and others, focuses attention on demanding jobs that are carried out under similar conditions (irregular schedules, quick response, field operations, unpredictable circumstances, system abuse) for similar stakes (life-and-death responsibilities, uncertain outcomes, personal danger, burnout). Finally, the difficulty of establishing social systems to handle emergency medical services points to the need for a new concept, *structural lag,* to refer to institutional defensiveness with regard to new programs. Resistance to change is not simply a result of ignorance or traditionalism in the face of technological development, as is implied by the term "cultural lag." Rather, such resistance is often due to distinct self-interests that prevent existing institutions from supporting any goals, however desirable, that might compromise the institutions' present advantages.

Third, the study points to specific research questions that could have a significant bearing on general theory. (1) It hints that mixed-gender ambulance teams might enhance communications with patients and perhaps even reduce aggressive responses. This possibility raises the question of whether mixed race, or language, or ethnicity teams might have beneficial effects on client-centered services, and, in general terms, of what are the interpersonal dynamics of transactions between mixed provider teams and clients. (2) In documenting the impact of abuse calls on public services, the study implies a need for more research on the social, political, and economic bases of misuse (false alarms, ambushes, shit calls). In particular, we need to know more about the assumed inverse relation between socioeconomic class and misuse of services, since some studies show nearly equal rates of misuse across the classes. In general, we need to know more about class differences in determining the proper use of public services. (3) As is true of the health care sector as a rule, the study of patient outcomes is not far advanced in ambulance work. More research about the impact on the patient's health status of different levels of attendant care would provide a basis for evaluating provider qualifications, for estimating the costs of employee turnover, and for comparing emergency medical services with other kinds of medical care. A study of outcomes could at the same time contribute to an improvement of ambulance operations and to our understanding of how institutions legitimate themselves on the basis of relatively little evidence. (4) The study emphasizes the ethical dilemma of an EMT whose formal responsibilities obligate him to resuscitate a dying patient who has apparently reached a natural end to life. Further research might reveal how treatment of the dying in other sectors of the health care field could be applied to ambulance work and, more generally, how unresolved value conflicts (about death) in our heterogeneous culture influence routine institutional operations. (5) Finally, considerations of the costs and benefits of ambulance services raise questions about the public's attitudes both toward the services and toward the life-style they entail. Researchers, perhaps using the approach called risk analysis, could investigate the hypothesis that rather than ambulances following a need, their availability might stimulate people to take more risks. Ambulance services may be part of a positive feedback loop that increases the need for such services. Although this study has many additional implications for sociology, these few will suffice to establish the point.

If these closing comments can usefully be drawn together into one general conclusion, it is this: ambulance work can be done properly only by dedicated workers who have the support of their superiors and the cooperation of the other components of the EMS system. Many EMS systems fail to meet one or more of these conditions (Metropolis certainly did), and the quality of patient care probably suffers because of it. At the same time, there are a great many committed EMTs and paramedics (at Liberty and elsewhere) who are struggling mightily to overcome unnecessarily difficult conditions in carrying out their work. As structures slowly change and as ambulance work becomes more institutionalized, perhaps it will be easier for these people to exercise their talents. Until then, may each of us find such people beneath the beacon should the siren sound for us.

notes to the text

Notes for Chapter 1

1. A useful statistical survey of the conditions of emergency medical services at the end of the 1960s can be found in John Camden, *Emergency Medical Services* (Westport, Conn.: Technomic Publishing Company, 1972).

2. The editors, "NREMT Surveys Completed," *Registry* (official publication of the National Registry of Emergency Medical Technicians) 9 (Autumn, 1979):5.

3. *The American Heritage Dictionary of the English Language,* William Morris, ed. (Boston: Houghton Mifflin, 1969), p. 41.

4. Katherine Traver Barkley, *The Ambulance: The Story of Emergency Transportation of Sick and Wounded Through the Centuries* (Hicksville, N.Y.: Exposition Press), p. 15. This book, though lacking structure, adequate references, critical capacity, and an index, does provide some interesting leads, a variety of illustrations, and a useful bibliography.

5. Ibid., pp. 61-73.

6. One of the most influential reports was *Accidental Death and Disability: The Neglected Disease of Modern Society* (Washington, D.C.: National Academy of Sciences—National Research Council, 1966).

7. Congressional hearings, *Emergency Medical Services Act of 1972,* Part I, Serial No. 92-83 (Washington, D.C.: U.S. Government Printing Office, 1972), p. 50.

8. Robert H. Kennedy, "What It Takes To Organize for Service," *The Modern Hospital* 106 (1966):1.

9. Julian A. Waller, "Rural Emergency Care—Problems and Prospects," *American Journal of Public Health* 63 (1973): 631-634.

10. Congressional hearings, EMS Act of 1972, p. 97.

11. American Hospital Association, *Emergency Medical Communications Systems* (Chicago: American Hospital Association, 1973), pp. 29-30.

12. Alfred M. Sadler, Jr., Blair L. Sadler, and Samuel B. Webb, Jr., *Emergency Medical Care: The Neglected Public Service* (Cambridge, Mass.: Ballinger, 1977), p. 7.

13. Camden, *Emergency Medical Services,* p. 67.

14. Committee on Injuries, American Academy of Orthopaedic Surgeons, *Emergency Care and Transportation of the Sick and Injured* (Chicago: American Academy of Orthopaedic Surgeons, 1971). The academy's Committee on Allied Health issued a second edition, revised, in 1977.

15. American Hospital Association, *Emergency Medical Communications Systems,* p. 19.

16. John J. Hanlon, "Emergency Medical Care as a Comprehensive System," *HSMHA Health Reports* 88 (1973): 581.

17. For a listing of diverse publications on ambulances covering the 1965-1977 period, see Joseph Lee Cook, *Ambulance Services: A Selected Bibliography* (Monticello, Ill.: Council of Planning Librarians, 1978). For some firsthand observations of ambulance operations about this time, see Dorothy Jean Douglas, "Occupational and Therapeutic Contingencies of Ambulance Services in Metropolitan Areas," dissertation, University of California, Davis, 1969; and Jack D.

Douglas, "Drug Crisis Intervention," Report to the National Commission on Mari-
huana and Drug Abuse, mimeograph (LaJolla: Department of Sociology, University of California, San Diego, undated), pp. 188-261. James O. Page provides a
detailed and vivid, as well as illustrated, recent history of EMS development in the
United States in *The Paramedics* (Morristown, N.J.: Backdraft Publications,
1979).

18. Congressional hearings, *EMS Act of 1972*, p. 31.
19. Camden, *Emergency Medical Services,* pp. 65-72.
20. National Academy of Sciences, *Accidental Death and Disability.*
21. National Academy of Sciences—National Research Council, *Roles and
Resources of Federal Agencies in Support of Comprehensive Emergency Systems*
(Washington, D.C.: Division of Medical Sciences, Committee on Emergency
Medical Services, 1972), pp. 14-20.
22. See, for example, Hanlon, *Emergency Medical Care as a Comprehensive
System,* p. 580; and Julius A. Roth, "Utilization of the Hospital Emergency
Department," *Journal of Health and Social Behavior* 12 (1971): 312-320.
23. American Hospital Association, *Emergency Medical Communications Sys-
tems,* p. 9.
24. Henry C. Huntley, "Legislation in Emergency Medical Services," in *Emergency Medical Care,* J. Clifford Findeiss, ed. (New York: Intercontinental Medical
Book Corporation, 1974), p. 249.
25. Sadler, Sadler, and Webb, *Emergency Medical Care: The Neglected Public
Service,* pp. 12-13.
26. Ibid., p. 16.
27. Comptroller General, *Progress, But Problems in Developing Emergency
Medical Service Systems,* Report to Congress, HRD-76-150 (Washington, D.C:
U.S. General Accounting Office, 1976), p. i, cover note.
28. Ibid., p. 2.
29. Sadler, Sadler, and Webb, *Emergency Medical Care: The Neglected Public
Service,* p. 20.
30. Ibid., p. 7, and Congressional Hearings, EMS Act of 1972, p. 81.
31. "Quantitative Status—Basic Level, *Registry 9* (Autumn 1979): 7.
32. Congressional hearings, EMS Act of 1972, pp. 125-130.
33. Committee on Allied Health, American Academy of Orthopaedic Surgeons, *Emergency Care and Transportation of the Sick and Injured,* 2nd ed. (Chicago: American Academy of Orthopaedic Surgeons, 1977), pp. 82-83. Although
this is a common description of what happens, the actual physiological process is
more complicated. See Eileen Courtes, "Brain Resuscitation Update," *Emergency*
13 (August 1981):48-49.
34. Division of Vital Statistics, Public Health Service, "Deaths and Death Rates
for Selected Causes," *The World Almanac and Book of Facts,* 1978 (New York:
Newspaper Enterprise Association, 1978), p. 953.
35. American Hospital Association, *Emergency Medical Communications Systems.*
36. National Safety Council, *Accident Facts* (Chicago: National Safety Council, 1972); National Academy of Sciences, *Accidental Death and Disability.*

37. Walter S. Graf, Sandra S. Polin, and Bertha L. Paegel, "A Community Program for Emergency Cardiac Care: A Three-Year Coronary Ambulance-Paramedic Evaluation," *Journal of the American Medical Association* 226 (1973): 156-160; N. M. White, et al., "Mobile Coronary Care Provided by Ambulance Personnel, " *British Medical Journal* 3 (1973): 618-622.

38. Hanlon, *Emergency Medical Care as a Comprehensive System.*

39. A. S. Freese, "Trauma: The Neglected Epidemic," *Saturday Review* 55 (May 13, 1972):35-37. The editors, "Improving Emergency Medical Services," *New England Journal of Medicine* 290 (1974): 628-629; Hanlon, *Emergency Medical Care as a Comprehensive System*; Huntley, "Legislation in EMS"; Waller, "Rural Emergency Care."

40. "Improving EMS"; Waller, "Rural Emergency Care."

41. John M. Waters and Carl H. Wells, "The Effects of a Modern Emergency Medical Care System in Reducing Automobile Crash Deaths," *The Journal of Trauma* 13 (1973): 645-647.

42. David R. Boyd, K. D. Mains, and B. A. Flashner, "A Systems Approach to Statewide Emergency Medical Care," *The Journal of Trauma* 13 (1973): 276-284.

43. George W. Baker, "Preventing Disastrous Behavior," in *Man and Society in Disaster*, G. W. Baker and Dwight W. Chapman, eds. (New York: Basic Books, 1962), p. 405.

44. Marc LeLonde, "The Canadian Health Care System—Its Impact on the Health of the Society," in *Medicine in a Changing Society*, Lawrence Corey, Michael F. Epstein, and Steven E. Saltman, eds., 2nd ed. (Saint Louis: C. V. Mosby Company, 1977); Ivan Illich, *Medical Nemesis: The Expropriation of Health* (New York: Bantam Books, 1976).

45. B. Latane and J. M. Darley, "Group Inhibition of Bystander Intervention in Emergencies," *Journal of Personality and Social Psychology* 10 (1968): 215-221.

46. P. Lipman, "Can You Afford to Be a Good Samaritan . . . Yes!" *RN* 37 (1974): 90-91.

47. Lowell S. Levin, Alfred H. Katz, and Erik Holst, *Self Care: Lay Initiatives in Health* (New York: Prodist, 1976).

48. Neighborhood Health Collectives of West Philadelphia, *Emergency Care and Other Good Ideas* (Philadelphia: A Movement for a New Society, 1974).

49. James V. Warren, "The Fireman Medic Lives up to His TV Image," *Medical Opinion* 5 (1976): 15-28.

50. Trevor Hughes, "The Choking Controversy," *Emergency* 11, no. 6 (June 1979): 34-41.

51. Emergency Department Nurses Association, "Greater Public Involvement Needed in Emergency Care Planning," *The Roadrunner* 3, no. 5 (September/October 1974): 3; Paul V. Joliet, "Development of Community Emergency Medical Services Councils," *Emergency Medicine Today* (August 1972): 26.

52. J. Clifford Findeiss, ed., *Emergency Medical Care* (New York: Intercontinental Medical Book Corporation, 1974), p. xi.

53. Don M. Benson, letter to the editor, *Journal of the American Medical Association* 225 (1973): 1527.

54. The editors, "Improving Emergency Medical Services," *New England Journal of Medicine*, p. 628; Anonymous, "The Economics of Highway Emergency Ambulance Services," *Northwest Medicine* 69 (1969): 333–338.

55. Roth, "Utilization of the Hospital Emergency Department."

56. Warren points out that the more affluent are inclined to contact their personal physician first in an emergency and that the time loss and the physician's lack of emergency training are detrimental to the victim's survival. Warren, "The Fireman Medic," p. 27.

57. A study in Milwaukee, where the "911" number was not in effect, found that only 5 percent of the adults polled knew how to call an ambulance. Peggy A. Knoebel, "Public Knowledge Regarding Emergency Telephone Numbers," unpublished research report, Department of Sociology, Anthropology, and Social Work, Marquette University, 1978.

58. It is significant that recent textbooks in medical sociology give little attention to the subject of emergency medical care. Only Twaddle and Hessler make explicit references to "emergency medical services" and "emergency medical technicians." Foster and Anderson make a passing mention of "ambulance crews" in connection with a digression on "emergency rooms," a subject treated more fully by Mechanic and by Denton. Mechanic, Robertson and Heagarty, and Enos and Sultan discuss the terms "accident" and "trauma," but only as classifications of morbidity and mortality rates and with no attention to the medical care mechanisms involved. There are no index listings for any of these terms in Susser and Watson, Coe, or Cockerham. William C. Cockerham, *Medical Sociology* (Englewood Cliffs, N.J.: Prentice-Hall, 1978); Rodney M. Coe, *Sociology of Medicine,* 2nd ed. (New York: McGraw-Hill, 1978); John A. Denton, *Medical Sociology* (Boston: Houghton Mifflin, 1978); Darryl D. Enos and Paul Sultan, *The Sociology of Health Care* (New York: Praeger, 1977); George M. Foster and Barbara Gallatin Anderson, *Medical Anthropology* (New York: John Wiley and Sons, 1978); David Mechanic, *Medical Sociology,* 2nd ed. (New York: The Free Press, 1978); Leon S. Robertson and Margaret C. Heagarty, *Medical Sociology* (Chicago: Nelson Hall, 1975); M. W. Susser and W. Watson, *Sociology in Medicine,* 2nd ed. (London: Oxford University Press, 1971); Andrew C. Twaddle and Richard M. Hessler, *A Sociology of Health* (St. Louis: C. V. Mosby, 1977).

59. A comparison of a few sources related to emergency medical services demonstrates the inconsistent terminology. For the basic level EMT, we can find listings of EMT, EMTA, EMT-1, EMT-1A, EMT-A, EMT-NA, REMT, REMTA, and EMT-Basic; for the advanced level, MICP, EMT-2, EMT-T, EMT-3, REMT-Paramedic, EMT-Paramedic, REMTA/P, and Paramedic. While there is a rationale behind each of these designations, different groups emphasize different rationales, and terms common in California, for example, might not be recognized on the East Coast. The sources used in this comparison were Alan B. Gazzangia, Lloyd T. Iseri, and Martin Baren, *Emergency Care: Principles and Practices for the EMT-Paramedic* (Reston, Va.: Reston Publishing Company, 1979); *Registry,* Fall 1979; *Emergency* 11, no. 9 (September 1979). The lack of institutionalization can also be seen in the fact that the use of the "star of life," the asterisk-like symbol of emergency medical services, is not at this time strictly defined or standardized. The editors, "DOT Paper Urges National Standards," *Registry,* Fall 1979: 4.

Notes for Chapter 2

1. "Initial Patient Survey" (mimeo), Tri-County Emergency Medical Services Council, Lansing, Michigan, 1974.
2. A comprehensive survey may require as many as 75 distinct observations. See "Initial Patient Survey." The primary purpose of this procedure is to assess the victim of severe trauma, such as that resulting from a fall or an automobile accident, where the injuries may be many, obscure, and potentially life-threatening. Because most emergency runs do not involve this kind of severe trauma, the value of a comprehensive survey is obvious in only a minority of runs. Though it may be recommended in theory, it is only selectively applied in practice, very much like the physician's reservation of a complete physical examination or a thorough medical history for certain cases.
3. The patient and his family will, of course, be asked to go over the same ground in the hospital, probably several times. But the hospital staff is constrained neither by the panic of the family, whom they have separated from the patient, nor by the feelings of the emergency service personnel, whose status in medical matters is regarded as unquestionably inferior. Indeed the reports filled out by ambulance personnel are often ignored by the medical staff, though admitting clerks find them useful as a source of personal data on the patient.
4. Nicholas Guild, *The Summer Soldier* (New York: Seaview Books, 1978), pp. 65-66. A study of the medical evaluation of patients in mental hospitals found a similar a priori method at work. "Once a person is designated abnormal, all of his other behaviors and characteristics are colored by that label. . . . The perception of his circumstances was shaped entirely by the diagnosis." D. L. Rosenhan, "On Being Sane in Insane Places," *Science* 179 (January 19, 1973): 250-258.
5. The techs' judgment in this area is supported by a classic study of the influence of culture on the response to pain: Mark Zborowski, "Cultural Components in Responses to Pain," *Journal of Social Issues* 8 (1952): 16-30. EMTs also come to realize that patients differ in the words they use to describe the same or similar conditions. David Mechanic uses the suggestive term "vocabularies of distress" to refer to this phenomenon. *Medical Sociology,* 2nd ed. (New York: The Free Press, 1978), p. 264.

Notes for Chapter 3

1. The office staff of the company is mainly female and over thirty, and the company has used female and nonwhite dispatchers. However, the personnel who work "on the cars" are likely to be young, white males.
2. Epinephrine (also called adrenalin) is a hormone, produced by the adrenal gland, that increases the strength and rate and effectiveness of cardiac contractions. It is used as an adjunct to electrical defibrillation (when the heart's contractions are weak and unproductive) and in asystole (when the heart is completely stopped). See, for example, Anthony S. Manoguerra, "Drug capsule: Epineph-

rine," *Emergency* 11 (November 1979): 31. In the incident that Jase recounts the drug was applied by a needle inserted under the rib cage and into the heart itself.

3. The body has been described as having a "biological clock" that synchronizes internal rhythms with the body's environment. Among the bodily processes that have been found to operate in cycles are the digestive process, body temperature, liver functions, cell division, heartbeat, secretion of such hormones as adrenalin, sensitivity to drugs, tolerance of pain, renal functions and urine output, epileptic seizures, sleep-wakefulness, and the ability to clear alcohol and drugs from the blood. For a general account of these matters, see John D. Palmer, *An Introduction to Biological Rhythms* (New York: Academic Press, 1976); and Gay Gaer Luce, *Body Time, Physiological Rhythms and Social Stress* (New York: Random House, 1971).

4. The body can eventually adjust to alterations in schedule, but this requires at least three to four days for some rhythms, seven to ten days for most, and two weeks or more for others. Geraldine Felton, "Body Rhythm Effects on Rotating Work Shifts," *Journal of Nursing Administration* (March-April 1975): 16-19.

5. For example, see Felton, "Body Rhythm Effects"; Grace Fass, "Sleep, Drugs, and Dreams," *American Journal of Nursing* 71 (December 1971): 2316-2320; and Palmer, *An Introduction to Biological Rhythms,* pp. 138, 153-157, 173. There is some evidence that depression and even industrial accidents are related to disturbances in biological rhythms. Reimer Lund, "Personality Factors and Desynchronization of Circadian Rhythms," *Psychosomatic Medicine* 36 (May-June 1974): 224-228.

6. For a recent account of the conditions of night work and for references on the subject, see Howard Robboy, "At Work with the Night Worker," in *Social Interaction,* Howard Robboy, Sidney L. Greenblatt, and Candace Clark, eds. (New York: St. Martin's Press, 1979), pp. 365-377.

7. At least two EMTs built up so much hostility toward the company that, as a final act of defiance, they quit with no notice—after having made arrangements for another job. Three times, to my knowledge, the company fired EMTs suddenly. Although in all these instances it was clear to nearly everyone that a break was inevitable, the timing of the event was always unexpected.

8. Discussions of reciprocity in social groups can be found in Alvin W. Gouldner, "The Norm of Reciprocity," *American Sociological Review* 25 (April 1960): 161-178; George C. Homans, *Social Behavior: Its Elementary Forms,* rev. ed. (New York: Harcourt Brace Jovanovich, 1974); and Peter M. Blau, *Exchange and Power in Social Life* (New York: John Wiley & Sons, 1964).

9. Claude Lévi-Strauss in his analysis of cross-cousin marriage distinguishes between "mutual" reciprocity and "universal" reciprocity, the former occurring between specific individuals and the latter involving indirect exchanges of favors within a network of three or more people. See Claude Lévi-Strauss, *The Elementary Structures of Kinship* (Boston: Beacon Press, 1969). The ambulance workers' informal norms about "covering" for each other—for meals, personal errands, and open shifts—is an excellent example of an "extended network" of reciprocity in contemporary society. Richard M. Emerson, however, distinguishes between exchange networks in structured exchange systems and in groups, and refers to "reciprocal altruism." See his paper "Social Exchange Theory," in *Annual Review*

of Sociology, Vol. 2, Alex Inkeles, James Coleman, and Neil Smelser, eds. (Palo Alto, Calif.: Annual Reviews, 1976), pp. 335-362.

10. The origins and operations of a sense of balanced reciprocity in exchange relations have been analyzed by Homans under the rubrics "the Aggression-Approval Proposition" and "Distributive Justice" (*Social Behavior,* pp. 37-40, 241-268), and by Blau, who uses the concept of "fair exchange" (*Exchange and Power,* pp. 156-157).

11. The crews and the owners make estimates of the relative inconvenience of covering. Tangible signs of commitment to an event or the involvement of other people weigh heavily in their estimation. Someone who has bought tickets for a concert would not be expected to come in; someone who merely has a date is less secure (depending on who the date is) but would be approached only in the most serious circumstances. A person planning simply to take it easy would be in a precarious situation and undoubtedly would be approached first.

12. In most cases the other city ambulance companies could cover Liberty's assigned zone if all Liberty's ambulances were making runs. Indeed, mechanical failures sometimes force an ambulance out of operation for an extended time, and the company's work is still handled adequately. However, the crews are aware that being short a car requires them to operate hurriedly at times and to call too often for backup from other companies. The crews associate these inefficiences with a reduction in the quality of care and thus interpret them as an undesirable condition rather than as a sign that the service can be handled with fewer cars. It is also possible that demonstrating the adequacy of fewer cars could threaten jobs, though I heard no talk of this.

13. This disjunction between work and family life was clearly expressed by a printer quoted in a famous study of the International Typographical Union: "Night workers don't have to punch the family time clock." Seymour Martin Lipset, Martin Trow, and James Coleman, *Union Democracy* (Garden City, N.Y.: Doubleday, 1962), p. 155.

14. The *Union Democracy* study, which gave considerable attention to social relations among workers, described this condition as follows: "Finally the night work (and most printers work night shifts for at least part of their careers) tends to increase printers' associations with each other. It reduces printers' opportunities to associate with nonprinters or to take part in neighborhood activities and mass entertainment; early in a man's career, it habituates him to occupation-linked leisure activities and releases him from the pressure of regular family life." Ibid., p. 158.

15. A notice on the Station 2 bulletin board on St. Christopher Hospital's letterhead read:

> **TO:** Liberty
> **FROM:** St. Chris' E.R. Admitting
> **DATE:** 7/15/78
> **SUBJECT:** Picnic

Hi,

How would you like to go to a picnic? We're planning a picnic for 8/16/78. We want you to come. Everyone bring what you want to eat & drink!

It's at Whitecliff Park, just off Highway 82, just past the state preserve. We'll be there at 10:00 A.M. You can come when you want. Just look for the St. Chris' signs. If you have any bats, balls, gloves, volleyballs, etc. bring them.
Hope to see you there.

16. A "front" is the idealized image of motives, means, and manners that an individual (or a group) wants outsiders to associate with him (or them). Dorothy J. Douglas uses the concept in describing how ambulance companies attempted to convince her (the researcher) that their operations were more impressive than was actually the case. See her article, "Managing Fronts in Observing Deviance," in *Research on Deviance*, Jack Douglas, ed. (New York: Random House, 1972), pp. 93-115.

17. We expect people to behave properly, therefore it is not remarkable when most of them do. What is remarkable is the blatant violation of our expectations. Thus, we recognize and remember the betrayals of the common code of behavior, while we allow the all but unanimous support of that code to pass unnoticed. Although infrequently, the EMTs do relate stories about the courtesy, kindness, and courage of patients and their families. For example, one of the crews was affected by the behavior of a young girl of about eight. As they told it, while the mother teetered on the edge of hysteria, complaining about being too weak to move, the inadequacies of her separated husband, the hostility of the neighbors, and her miserably bad luck, the little girl took over the management of the home. She comforted her mother, found misplaced items, telephoned to make arrangements for herself, and handled everything with unbelievable maturity and good humor. The EMTs were noticeably moist around the eyes as they described the scene.

18. Debriefing is the questioning of an agent to obtain information gathered on a mission. Commonly used by the military and by intelligence agencies, the term was popularized in reports on the astronaut programs and has by now become part of the public vocabulary.

19. Learning the folklore within the company seems to be similar to Sudnow's "counting deaths" in the hospital. David Sudnow, *Passing On: The Social Organization of Dying* (Englewood Cliffs, N.J.: Prentice-Hall, 1967), pp. 36-42.

20. Being forced to pace one's efforts according to the demands of outsiders is not unique; ambulance personnel share this condition with many other workers. Even such high-status workers as physicians must respond to the bidding of their "beepers" or of public address systems. However, while ambulance workers must be prepared to swing into action immediately, higher status workers can arrange to have barriers placed between themselves and the source of the demands. Stanley Milgram in "The Experience of Living in Cities" (*Science,* March 13, 1970: 1461-1468) lists a variety of techniques commonly used to control the flood of demands and to prevent what he calls "system overload." Secretaries, receptionists, and answering services give physicians control over when, and how, they respond. Alan E. Nourse's novel, *The Practice* (New York: Harper & Row, 1978), is a physician's fictional account of, among other things, how professionals can insulate themselves even against the demands of their group practice colleagues.

21. Occasionally there are complications in interpreting this rule. If two crews already in quarters have been making emergency runs and a third returns from errands, there are grounds for claiming the third crew should make the next run. Or if one has handled three calls while the others have had one each, the first may claim the right to be last car out.

22. Ambulance services handle meal periods in different ways. Employees of the company grumbled about not having a policy that guarantees a protected meal-time. They claim that other private companies allow each crew time to eat and will even "give away" calls, that is, refer them to another company, rather than disturb an out-of-service crew. On the other hand, it is never easy for first responders assigned to cover a particular sector to shift their responsibility to other units. They are likely to have to eat on the run. A report on the emergency medical system in Baltimore, for example, features a picture of a fire department paramedic having a quick lunch in the back of his ambulance. See Joe Calderone, "With Ambulance No. 7: A Ride on the Wild Side," *Baltimore News American,* June 23, 1980, p. 1A.

23. Two examples should clarify this point. Those who have tried to pursue hobbies in quarters, such as building model airplanes or painting ceramics, have inevitably become discouraged because of the problem of dealing with paint brushes and partially glued pieces when a call comes in. Those who have tried to study in quarters—chemistry, German, flight instruction, electrocardiogram inter-pretation—agree that it is difficult to accomplish anything even during a slow shift.

24. Several conditions support the five finger discount. First, there is loose con-trol over the dispensing of exhaustible supplies. Ironically, a state of trust among workers contributes to this condition, as does inefficient organization. Second, administrative divisions among the components of the Emergency Medical Ser-vices System (hospitals, fire department, and ambulance companies) encourage both organizational inefficiencies and pseudoadversary relations. Third, govern-ment financing of part of the system provides an excuse for violators to argue that the supplies belong to all the citizens. Fourth, extensive volunteer EMS work by personnel, as in the case where urban and suburban or rural systems are separate, provides motivation for "lifting" supplies. Dorothy Jean Douglas found a similar kind of on-the-job theft from hospitals in the companies she studied. However, she also noted instances of an ambulance company owner instructing his employees to steal and of hospital personnel looking favorably on lifting in some cases. See Douglas's dissertation, *Occupational and Therapeutic Contingencies of Ambulance Services in Metropolitan Areas* (Ann Arbor, Michigan: University Microfilms, 1970), pp. 92-94, 183-185, 221.

25. Many of the people in this EMS system are uncertain about even routine procedures. Several times, nurses, who were asked for replacement supplies for an ambulance, queried the crews to make sure the ambulance company would not charge the patients for these supplies anyway. Once assured that the company would charge only a flat fee, the nurses turned over the supplies. This uncertainty may be explained by the fact that, when I was working at Station 2, the system had been operating for less than a year. Another explanation derives from the difficulty of communicating across the boundaries of the several organizations the system comprises. For more on this, see Chapter 7, "Accidental Relations."

Notes for Chapter 4

1. Dorothy Jean Douglas describes the hiring practices and job requirements of a private ambulance company on the West Coast in the 1960s. See her dissertation, *Occupational and Therapeutic Contingencies of Ambulance Services in Metropolitan Areas* (Ann Arbor, Michigan: University Microfilms, 1970), pp. 74-85.

2. According to a survey by the National Registry of Emergency Medical Technicians (NREMT): "Although the EMT is one of the newer members of the allied health team, the study shows that the occupation ranks second in total numbers nationally certified, exceeded only by medical technologists." This news account does not say what proportion of EMTs are nationally certified, or how that proportion compares with those of the other thirty-seven occupations licensed by the thirteen agencies responding to the survey. *Registry* (not dated but about September 1979): 5.

3. Suburban Features, for example, in 1979 provided a syndicated supplement that stated: "If you have thought about working in surgery, wrestling with medical emergencies or managing patients on a daily basis, you don't have to become a doctor to do so. For instance, when the surgeon calls 'scalpel', it is the surgical technologist who responds. Medical emergencies also are all in a day's work for the emergency medical technicians or paramedics. . . ." "Health Jobs Come in All Places," *Milwaukee Journal,* October 24, Supplement on careers, pp. 12-13. As of 1979 there were approximately 270,000 EMTs and EMT-Ps (paramedics) in the United States. The Department of Labor projects a need for at least 100,000 more to be trained by 1990. See "NAEMT Presents Testimony on EMS Act," *The EMT Newsletter,* no. 3 (April 1979): 8. *The Occupational Outlook Handbook,* 1978-79 edition, published by the Bureau of Labor Statistics of the U.S. Department of Labor (Washington, D.C.: U.S. Government Printing Office, 1978), includes a section describing EMTs (pp. 473-476).

4. "Periodicals Related to EMS," *JEMS: A Journal of Emergency Medical Services* 5, no. 1 (March 1980): 22-29.

5. "Transition," *Newsweek,* June 9, 1980, p. 106

6. See Chapter 1, note 59.

7. See Chapter 1, note 58.

8. The petition disappeared from the service station as soon as company personnel pointed out to the station owner the contradiction in his policy. The drive itself had no chance of success because the police department could not satisfy the federal standards for EMS personnel or equipment. The drive showed how little the public understood about the character of the new emergency medical services.

9. Estimates in 1979 were that of 262,000 current EMTs and EMT-Ps (paramedics), 60 percent were citizens who volunteered their time for training and for active duty. "NAEMT Presents Testimony on EMS Act," *The EMT Newsletter* 3 (April 1979): 3, 5, 8.

10. See S. Vahovich, *'73 Profile of Medical Practice* (Chicago: American Medical Association, 1973). The proportion of women in medical school has been increasing, however, and by the late 1970s about 25 percent of the first-year

classes were women. See Travis L. Gordon, "Study of U.S. Medical School Applicants 1977-1978," *Journal of Medical Education* 54, no. 9 (September 1979): 677-702.

11. See T. M. Ryan, "Some Current Trends in the Soviet Health Services," *The Medical Officer* 13 (February 1970): 83. Michael Swafford shows that health services in Russia receive lower compensation than other occupational categories in his article, "Sex Differences in Soviet Earnings," *American Sociological Review* 43, no. 5 (October 1978): 657-673.

12. Douglas describes the personnel of the private companies she studied as very low in educational and occupational attainment, and ambulance work as being a second or third choice even for many of them. *Occupational and Therapeutic Contingencies,* pp. 86-90.

13. The National Registry reported that through May 31, 1980, 142,738 candidates had passed the written section of their examinations and 24,520 had failed. "Quantitative Status—Basic Level," *Registry* 12, no. 2 (July 1980): 7. The coordinator for the EMT training program in Liberty's region said the class he was completing at the beginning of this study began with 127 students, but only 63 were prepared to take the final examination. He attributed the high drop-out rate in part to firefighters who had been pressured into taking the course and to young people who were attracted to the lights and sirens but weren't really interested in the medical aspects of the work. A coordinator in another region told her class that if they had a "C" average in the course they probably would not pass the National Registry exam. Only nine of fifteen students in her previous class had passed it, though sixteen of twenty-two had passed the state test.

14. Of the eighteen Liberty employees whose backgrounds are known to me, seven had finished or were finishing college and seven others had done coursework beyond the high school level. Thus 78 percent of them had done post-high school academic work. According to a 1978 report on EMT-Paramedic trainees, about 60 percent (though there are some discrepancies in the figures) had done post-high school work. See Harvey A. Siegal et al., "The EMT-Paramedic: A Profile of Voluntary Medical Paraprofessionals," *The EMT Journal* 2, no. 3 (September 1978): 50.

15. The ambulance service in Baltimore, Maryland, which is under the auspices of the fire department evidently suffers from the same morale problems. A high-ranking official says the firefighters shun ambulance work because (1) they lack the proper training and therefore are scared, (2) they would rather watch TV in the station than run all the time, and (3) the service retains a stigma from the time when it was common practice to detail the department's rejects to the ambulance service. Joe Calderone, "Personnel Shortage Threatens Service," *Baltimore News American,* June 22, 1980, p. 7A.

16. For example, Allan J. Mayer mentions policemen, garbage collectors, and ambulance drivers together when he anticipates the decamping of social service workers because of insufficient pay. "Inflation: A Doomsday Scenario," *Newsweek,* March 24, 1980,: 28.

17. Each rate was reported by someone in that specific occupation. Those EMTs who are paid as firefighters or policemen receive rates higher than any reported in the table.

18. "National Registry EMT Survey," *Registry* 10, no. 4 (December 1979): 6.
19. This is one of the themes stressed by Everett C. Hughes, *Men and Their Work* (Glencoe, Illinois: The Free Press, 1958), pp. 54-55, 88.
20. U.S. Bureau of the Census, "Detailed Occupation of the Experienced Civilian Labor Force and Employed Persons," *1970 Census of Population: Characteristics of the Populations* (Washington, D.C.: U.S. Government Printing Office, 1973). For an informative analysis of how the category of service workers has been constructed and what the label actually covers, see Chapters 16 and 20 in Harry Braverman's *Labor and Monopoly Capital: The Degradation of Work in the Twentieth Century* (New York: Monthly Review Press, 1974), pp. 359-374, 424-449.
21. The typology in Table 2 presents a rather prevalent, though arguable, conception of occupations. It is based on the discussions in Braverman, *Labor and Monopoly Capital;* Amitai Etzioni, ed., *The Semi-Professions and Their Organization* (New York: The Free Press, 1969); Harold L. Wilensky, "The Professionalization of Everyone?" *American Journal of Sociology* 70, no. 2 (September 1964): 137-158; and Everett Cherrington Hughes, "The Study of Occupations," in *Sociology Today: Problems and Prospects,* Robert K. Merton, Leonard Broom, and Leonard S. Cottrell, Jr., eds. (New York: Basic Books, 1959), pp. 442-458. Other frequently mentioned dimensions—the right to privileged communication, a code of ethics or of occupational norms, and the establishment of an occupation-based organization—were not included in the table because they do little to further distinctions among occupations.
22. An excellent analysis of "public service workers who interact directly with citizens in the course of their jobs, and who have substantial discretion in the execution of their work" is Michael Lipsky's book, *Street-Level Bureaucracy: Dilemmas of the Individual in Public Services* (New York: Russell Sage Foundation, 1980). Though the street-level bureaucrats with whom he is concerned are representatives of public services, his account applies in many ways to the employees of private ambulance companies.
23. Autonomy by default describes an occupation "left wholly to its own devices because there is no strong public concern with its work, because it works independently of any functional division of labor, and because its work (in complexity, specialization, or observability) precludes easy evaluation and control by others." Eliot Freidson, *Professional Dominance: The Social Structure of Medical Care* (New York: Atherton Press, 1970), p. 136. Freidson cites as examples nightclub magicians, circus acrobats, cab drivers, and lighthouse keepers. Everett C. Hughes uses the terms "power by default" and "mandate by default" to refer to a similar phenomenon, using as examples classroom teachers and "professional" criminals. Hughes, *Men and Their Work,* pp. 451-452.
24. Jack Olsen, *Night Watch* (New York: Times Books, 1979), p. 16.
25. Siegal et al. found that 78 percent of the paramedic trainees they surveyed had aspirations to health sector careers. "The EMT-Paramedic: A Profile," p. 52.
26. Of 42 employees, a minimum of 25 were involved in definite extracurricular EMS activities that were not compensated for in any but nominal ways. Information was not available on the other 17 employees in this regard.
27. Volunteer EMTs must bear all of the responsibility and the requirements of paid EMTs, but must do so while earning a livelihood and fitting training and runs

into spare time at their own expense. Donald L. Metz, "The Emergency Medical Services Volunteer," paper presented at the annual meeting of the Midwest Sociological Society, Minneapolis, April 16, 1977. Moreover, Thom Dick suggests that off-duty involvement in EMS may accelerate burnout and shorten EMT careers. See "Anxiety in the Street," *JEMS: A Journal of Emergency Medical Services* 5, no. 4 (June 1980): 29-31.

28. The content of the course can be seen in the widely used textbook *Emergency Care and Transportation of the Sick and Injured,* 2nd ed., revised (Chicago: American Academy of Orthopaedic Surgeons, 1977).

29. The following hypotheses will show what I mean. Where the training program is the responsibility of a dominant medical institution—hospital or medical school—physicians will play a large role in instruction. If the program is in a densely populated area or is the result of a collaboration of several medical institutions, the instructors are more likely to be paramedics. In sparsely populated areas or where volunteers organize the course, nonmedical (and nonparamedical) personnel will have greater involvement in instruction.

30. In this as in the rest of life necessity interprets the rules. Nurse James said the coordinator of an EMT course should have 25 hours of experience on an ambulance, but she was the only one available and willing to take the job. It was a case of compromise the standards or abandon the course altogether.

31. Frank Meister, Jr., et al., "Comparison of the Oral Hygiene and Periodontal Health Status of a Class of Dental Students: As Freshman and as Seniors," *Journal of Preventive Dentistry* 6 (1980): 245-252.

32. This term is discussed in Thomas J. Scheff, "Decision Rules, Types of Error, and Their Consequences in Medical Diagnosis," *Behavioral Science* 8 (1963): 97-107. Scheff uses the example of the medical rule "When in doubt, continue to suspect illness." The more specific of these informal norms are similar to what are called "treatment philosophies" by Kathleen Knafl and Gary Burkett in "Professional Socialization in a Surgical Speciality: Acquiring Medical Judgment," *Social Science and Medicine* 9 (1975): 397-404.

33. An example of the explicit statement of this decision rule is the following; "It is essential that rescuers *overreact* and *overtreat* in cases where spinal injury is suspected. They should approach each accident as though the worst had happened and suspect spinal injury even with what may appear as only minor trauma." (Italics in the original.) Lou Jordan and Denise Calabrese, "Treating Spinal Cord Injuries," *Emergency* 12, no. 6 (June 1980): 42.

34. The written examinations from the National Registry and from the states seem to be well protected. Usually coordinators will base their general advice on their experience from previous years. Occasionally, however, the same tests will be used for several courses in a row, in which case the coordinators may have specific information to pass along.

35. The term comes from Joseph Heller's novel, *Catch-22* (New York: Simon and Schuster, 1961).

36. This situation occurs frequently in occupations where the route into particular jobs is closely controlled. For example, one must have seaman's papers to take a job on a working vessel, but the papers are only available to someone who has

such a job. Or again, one cannot work in certain places without a union card, but in order to get a union card one must have a job there.

37. The procedures for the EMT-Intermediate (EMT-I) status include a description of how the field experience provisions can be handled for National Registry certification. "New Certification Level Gains Approval," *The EMT Journal* 4, no. 3 (September 1980): 83–84.

38. Knafl and Burkett observed that though the process of decision making prior to treatment was highly institutionalized in an orthopedic surgical residency program, there was no such institutionalization of subsequent evaluative processes. "Professional Socialization," p. 401. The enactment in the late 1970s of new regulations for the relicensing of physicians, dentists, nurses, and others was a belated recognition of the need for quality control even among the elite professionals. The editors of *Registry* reported (Fall 1979: 5) that fewer than one-third of the allied health occupations they surveyed required recertification or continuing education.

39. The term was evidently coined by Victor Thompson in *Modern Organization* (New York: Knopf, 1961). The most influential discussion of the concept was that of Erving Goffman in *The Presentation of Self in Everyday Life* (Garden City, N.Y.: Doubleday, 1959). Most of his subsequent writings extend that discussion. Knafl and Burkett explain how the "gamesmanship" of a residency contributes to the professional socialization of the physicians by allowing them to practice acting like orthopedic surgeons and by developing their confidence. "Professional Socialization," p. 402.

40. One incident of many involved a hypoglycemic man in Martinsburg, West Virginia, who had been pronounced dead by the coroner but who was found to be breathing in a last-minute check of the body bag in a funeral home. United Press International, "Man Declared Dead Saved by Last-Minute Check," *Metropolitan Daily*, May 23, 1980, part 1, p. 3.

41. The ambiguities confronting the ambulance attendant are a milder form of the uncertainties the medical student and the physician must deal with. Renee C. Fox, "Training for Uncertainty," *Dominant Issues in Medical Sociology*, Howard D. Schwartz and Cary S. Kart, eds. (Reading, Mass.: Addison-Wesley, 1978).

42. Hughes, *Men and Their Work*, Chapter 6. Hughes suggests that guilty knowledge is an unavoidable part of the license granted to those occupations that receive society's mandate to control a part of the division of labor.

43. The idea of role-set has been usefully analyzed by Robert K. Merton, particularly in "The Role-Set: Problems in Sociological Theory," *British Journal of Sociology* 8 (1957): 106–120.

Notes for Chapter 5

1. The crews come to think of the rigs as having personalities; one is difficult to start, another inclined to stall, another has an unreliable radio or is accident-prone or is always in the shop. This outlook is described in a somewhat dramatic fashion in a novel by Hugh Miller. ". . . Dan McGoldrick, inclining more to an inherited streak of dark superstition, averred . . . that the ambulance was cursed. He could

bring forward precedents for his belief. There was a wagon in London that the men had finally refused to handle, because of its ominously poor record of service. People had died wholesale and the vehicle had even tried, once, to wipe out its driver. There was another in Scotland and one in Dublin. The nature of the work, Dan hinted, imposed a spiritual quality on the ambulance, and some of them did not have the in-built harmony required to do the job." *Ambulance* (New York: St. Martin's Press, 1975), p. 153.

2. The drivers have more difficulty than the techs in remembering patients, because their contact is not as intense or prolonged. Flash, who drives much of the time, will sometimes strain to recall whether he has handled a particular person before.

3. Much of the organization's concern that paperwork be handled properly has to do with defending against the possibility of litigation. This function of the trip report is emphasized in Kate Boyd, "The Power of Paperwork," *JEMS: A Journal of Emergency Medical Services* 5, no. 5 (July 1980): 20–27. The crews express the company's concern in more earthy language: "Well, you know how it is by now. When I signed on, Pete [one of the owners] told me there were two things to remember: 'Don't step on your own dick,' and 'Cover the Company's ass.' I guess that about says it."

4. It is impossible to say whether it was connected with her attitude toward paperwork, but the fact is that the owners grew unhappy with Jilly and eventually forced her out of the company, though they did not directly fire her.

5. The company does recognize that on certain runs the techs cannot be expected to handle the paperwork in routine fashion. Among the circumstances considered exceptional are serious accidents with multiple victims, runs that require CPR, and instances of unidentified patients who are unconscious or who speak a language the crews cannot translate. In these cases the office staff would attempt to track down the necessary information through the police department, the fire department, the hospital, and other sources. Few of the runs are so unambiguous, however; criticism centers on the more frequent cases where the tech gives more attention to the patient than the reported condition seems to warrant.

6. A complete view requires that we go beyond short-run interests. As the owners frequently point out, unless they can collect for the services they provide, there will be no services provided. In other words, the short-run benefit of the patients is ultimately best served by giving due regard to the long-run interests of the company and the EMS system, that is, by doing the paperwork. The paperwork makes it possible for the company to collect its fees and for the EMS system to maintain some kind of quality control.

7. This feature of ambulance work is equivalent to the "counting deaths" phenomenon Sudnow reported having observed among hospital workers. David Sudnow, *Passing On: The Social Organization of Dying* (Englewood Cliffs, N.J.: Prentice-Hall, 1967), pp. 36–42.

8. As the rate of turnover of personnel increases, it becomes more difficult for the crews to know each other well enough to come up with appropriate and convincing nicknames. At Liberty the trend is simply to use given names for newer employees, while older ones usually have more colorful labels.

9. Many private ambulance companies do only gerrie work; that is, they transport bodies, usually elderly ones, between home or nursing home and hospital.

Some of the Liberty attendants began with the company when it did only gerrie work and made the transition to street work when the company became part of the metropolitan EMS system. Brush seemed unable to make the transition.

10. Complaints about particular EMTs are carried up the line informally in most cases. This means the people who are friendly with the owners have a great deal of influence in determining the owners' opinions of attendants. However, there is evidence that the owners try to be fair. They do not base a dismissal on a single episode, and occasionally they survey the employees informally to determine the accuracy of reports.

11. See Vincente Navarro's work on the subject. A representative piece is "Women in Health Care," *New England Journal of Medicine* 202 (1975): 398-402.

12. A study in Michigan found that a large proportion of female attendants had romantic ties within their companies. Specifically, about one-third were married to men in the same ambulance company; probably many more were engaged or otherwise obligated. The authors conclude that long-term commitment to EMS is supported by these familial ties; they do not speculate about possible disruptions caused by sexual rivalry. Harry Perlstadt and Lola Jean Kozak, "Emergency Medical Services in Small Communities: Volunteer Ambulance Corps," *Journal of Community Health* 2, no. 3 (Spring 1977): 178-188.

13. Women evidently handle the work well in other places, too. See Joan Declaire, "AmCare's Women," *Emergency* 11, no. 7 (July 1979): 58-59, for some comments on an ambulance service in Oklahoma City.

14. Perhaps Barb was exaggerating when she claimed to be part of a two-person crew that moved a 400-pound DOE. She also recounts the story of a patient who was unruly in the back of the ambulance. She put her knee in his groin and leaned on it. He shouted, "Lady, you're bustin' my left nut!" She told him if he didn't behave she'd bust both of them, and it seemed to calm him down.

15. One way in which heterosexual relationships differ from homosexual ones is that the former can result in pregnancy. While this might create problems for the company, I never heard it specifically mentioned as a concern.

16. The company did not make any allowances to keep Jilly on the roster. Although she was recovering from an injury and had just married a fellow employee, she was told she would be required to work a full sixty-four-hour week and could not work on the same shift as her husband. The owners had not mentioned the no-spouse-on-the-same-shift rule earlier, even though they knew about the marriage plans. There were many relatives working in the company at that time. And there were many part-timers doing eight-hour stretches for less than forty hours a week.

17. After she left Liberty, Sonya worked for a while as an aide in a physician's office but told people she missed ambulance work. Her departure was apparently not prompted by lack of interest or the need for more money. Further, she maintained a romantic tie with one of the Liberty EMTs.

18. To some extent dispatchers are blamed for failures that are not their fault. Information transferred hurriedly through several excited people is not very reliable. Dispatchers have difficulty unscrambling the facts in many cases and sometimes add to the ambiguity by contributing their own interpretations. The ambiguity is not simply a result of incompetence but is largely an inevitable difficulty of the

event. The complaints are common. Hugh Miller makes a passing reference to it (*Ambulance,* p. 258): "They drove quickly to the address given by the police. As ever, the details had not been given very clearly. . . ."

19. Accidents occur constantly with the ambulances, but most of them are minor, and few, if any, involve people learning to drive hot. Vehicles in the repair shops are there for body work or routine mechanical maintenance. The few major crashes involve experienced drivers. The company's concern about scrapes and dents moved it to issue regulation 9.121: "Whenever an ambulance is backing up, the technician will be outside the car guiding the driver and watching for obstructions (unless there is a patient in the car, in which case the technician will be watching out the rear and side windows)."

20. Since most Liberty employees work from 48 to 72 hours per week, and since many of them live outside the city, the costs of their participating in these programs is not inconsiderable. A day-long seminar consumes half a weekend, and even a three-hour in-service takes a whole evening.

21. These figures assume there were 32 attendants on the roster (though hirings and firings caused fluctuations). The attendance at three meetings was 8 (25 percent), 12 (38 percent), and 17 (56 percent). The first was at a hospital; the other two were at Station 2 and included the six attendants on duty. The last was a meeting with the city's commissioner of health. The topics of in-services vary. These sessions were respectively on a hospital disaster plan, standards for using oxygen and suctioning equipment, and the coordination of the municipal EMS system.

22. Reports were checked on occasions when at least a dozen had accumulated (before they were taken to the main office), when the checking would not obtrude on activities in quarters, and when the checker was not tired, busy, or otherwise distracted. The researcher's reports were excluded, as were "no transports." The few DOEs were included, about half with the vitals recorded as zeros.

23. Some companies structure the regular evaluation of attendants' performances. The state agency claimed that it does not have sufficient staff to handle the enormous amount of paperwork involved in transcribing and analyzing data from EMT reports (which are forwarded to the agency anyway). It relies on certification and recertification of personnel and on periodic inspections of equipment as quality controls.

24. This characteristic of a low-status job is not uncommon. For example, Hessler and others have analyzed the blocked mobility of community health workers, which made them prisoners of their positions. See the accounts in W. Holton, P.K.-M. New, and R. M. Hessler, *Citizen Participation and Interagency Relations,* Research Report to the National Institute of Mental Health, Washington, D.C., 1972; and P.K.-M. New and R. M. Hessler, "Neighborhood Health Centers: Traditional Medical Care in an Outpost?" *Inquiry* 9 (1972): 45-58.

25. A few of the EMTs at Liberty have studied books on cardiac arrhythmias and drug effects irregularly. Others have attended weekend conferences and even learned the techniques of starting IVs. Still others have worked at jobs in related technologies—respiration therapy, physical therapy, lab technology, and as paramedics (perhaps at an intermediate level). It is not unreasonable to refer to these people as overtrained, since they have reason to feel they have pertinent skills and knowledge which they are not allowed to apply.

26. This approach emphasizes the stress response rather than the stress event or stimulus. Hans Selye, who first elaborated on the idea for health care, calls the physiological response "the stress syndrome" and the stressful agent the "stressor." See his article, "The Stress Syndrome," *American Journal of Nursing* 65, no. 3 (March 1965): 97–99. David Mechanic provides a good summary of the various conceptualizations of stress in *Medical Sociology*, 2nd ed. (New York: The Free Press, 1978), pp. 222–246.

27. Mike Olds, a Baltimore paramedic, reports similar signs: "After a 10-hour shift, when you go through with six or seven or ten nothing runs, like sick at home or a transport, you get back to the station and you say to hell with this place, what am I doing, I want to get out and go home." Olds then adds, "But the next morning, when you wake up and it's time to go in, you start to want it all over again. At least that's the way it is for me." Joe Calderone, "The Paramedics' Grinding Routine," *Baltimore News American*, June 23, 1980, p. 1A. Olds is 23 and has a resiliance his older colleagues, according to the account, seem to have lost.

28. This point is made clearly in H. Basowitz et al., *Anxiety and Stress* (New York: McGraw-Hill, 1955).

29. A widely circulated list of 130 stress-ranked occupations is based on admission records from community health centers in Tennessee. The original report, which analyzed the 30 most stressful occupations, is Michael J. Colligan, Michael J. Smith, and Joseph J. Hurrell, "Occupational Incidence Rates of Mental Health Disorders," *Journal of Human Stress* 3, no. 3 (September 1977): 34–39.

30. One can get an idea of the variety of definitions, components, and correlates of occupational stress or job stress from the articles in two collections: Lennart Levi, *Society, Stress, and Disease* (New York: Oxford University Press, 1971); and Alan McLean, *Occupational Stress* (Springfield, Ill.: Charles C. Thomas, 1974).

31. Robert D. Caplan et al., *Job Demands and Worker Health,* HEW Publication No. (NIOSH) 75-160 (Washington, D.C.: U.S. Government Printing Office, 1975). Of the twenty-three occupations included in this study, policemen were the most similar to ambulance workers with regard to job demands. Surprisingly, police were found to be relatively low in stress, perhaps due to the fact that they have more certain careers, greater opportunity to use their abilities, and better pay than ambulance workers.

32. This gradual change of attitude was noted by another Baltimore paramedic (see note 27 above): "I used to think everybody was really sick, and when we responded I treated them like they were sick. . . . But I'm not as sympathetic as I used to be, not after seeing as many people as I've seen, and after people being the way they are, calling us when they have a cold. . . . I don't know how long ago it was before I became cold toward people. . . . Now all I can think about is retiring and getting out of this place." Calderone, "The Paramedics' Grinding Routine," p. 4A. In a similar vein one of the Metropolis firefighter EMTs told some Liberty attendants he was transferring back to the fire crews because the rescue squad was getting to be too much the same thing.

33. This cynicism seems to be related to the lack of appreciation for their work that is seen in low pay, little authority, and lack of institutional support (i.e., no career ladder). It differs, therefore, from the cynicism ascribed to medical students and explained by their temporary adjustment to limited responsibility and the in-

creasingly technical emphasis of their clinical training. See Howard S. Becker and Blanche Geer, "The Fate of Idealism in Medical School," *American Sociological Review* 23 (1958): 50-56.

34. For a description of these characteristics, see Christine Maslack, "Burned-out," *Human Behavior* (1976): 16-22. For an excellent description of the conditions surrounding burnout in EMS work, see Nancy K. Graham, "Done in, Fed up, Burned out: Too Much Attrition in EMS," *JEMS: A Journal of Emergency Medical Services* 6, no 1 (January 1981): 24-29, and her companion article, "Part 2: How to Avoid a Short Career," *JEMS* 6, no. 2 (February 1981): 25-31.

35. Social workers, psychologists, counselors, teachers, and others are included in the study by Jerry Edelwich (with Archie Brodsky), *Burn-Out: Stages of Disillusionment in the Helping Professions* (New York: Human Sciences Press, 1980). The Maslack article cited above covers a similar range of occupations.

36. Joanne Giza points out that the families of the burned-out workers suffer, too. She describes her policeman husband as becoming "a closed, bitter, tense man. The job and its attendant stresses slowly drained the peace, the contentment and the joy from our lives. . . . The life that Jim saw and lived when he was on duty . . . invaded our home through his outbursts, his impatience, his silence, his separateness." "My Turn: A Policeman's Lot," *Newsweek,* November 14, 1980, p. 31.

37. A search for the oldest paramedic found at least one man active at age 57 and a slightly younger one who had been in EMS work in the street for 34 years. Neither was showing signs of paramedic burnout. "Still Doin' It," *Paramedics International* 4, no. 3 (Fall 1979): 41-42.

38. Even among the public EMS organizations turnover is being recognized as a serious problem. It is especially striking in a field where most of the employees are very young. See Graham, "Done in." Ray F. Reed discusses the reasons for turnover among Dallas fire department paramedics in "Job Satisfaction Survey of EMS Personnel," *The EMT Journal* 5, no. 1 (February 1981): 21-26. Robert Elling reports on a survey of paramedics in New York City in "Stress as Related to the EMT-P," *The EMT Journal* 4, no. 4 (December 1980): 32-34. He makes the interesting point that "the more dedicated, idealistic, and competent the EMT-P is, the greater the chances he will suffer the effects of stress."

39. A survey of occupational structures concluded that "education, experience, and job performance can hardly exert an impact on earnings or occupational status in sectors of the economy where institutional rules permit little advancement or specify identical wages." "Project Appropriations for 1979," *Russell Sage Foundation 1979* (New York: Russell Sage Foundation, 1980), p. 26. Thus the structure of the work sector (e.g., the lack of a job ladder) of which ambulance work is a part provides little incentive for the worker to improve his education, experience, or job performance.

40. The Liberty vote was not unusual. In fiscal 1979 unions won only 45 percent of the 8,043 representation elections conducted by the National Labor Relations Board. "Unions Lose More Often," *Metropolitan Daily,* July 28, 1980: Accent, p. 1.

41. It is not clear how worker input could be formalized in small organizations to correspond to the suggestion for large bureaucracies in Barry A. Stein and Rosa-

beth Moss Kanter, "Building the Parallel Organization: Creating Mechanisms for Permanent Quality of Work Life," *Journal of Applied Behavioral Science* 16, no. 3 (1980): 371–386.

Notes for Chapter 6

1. Graham considers the process to be a result of the anger directed toward patients by the providers suffering from burnout. Nancy K. Graham, "Done in, Fed up, Burned out: Too Much Attrition in EMS," *JEMS: A Journal of Emergency Medical Services* 6, no. 1 (January 1981): 29. My observations suggest that stereotyping is one of the EMT's techniques for preparing for a patient on a run, is inevitable in jobs with brief but direct client contacts, is grounded to some extent in experience, and thus is not simply a product of career-end fatigue. We can recognize that it is inevitable without denying that it is also unfair and at times harmful.

2. Roth points out that there is "no evidence that professional training succeeds in producing a universalistic moral neutrality. On the contrary, we are on much safer ground to assume that those engaged in dispensing professional services (or any other services) will apply the evaluations of social worth common to their culture and will modify their services with respect to those evaluations *unless discouraged from doing so by the organizational arrangements under which they work.*" (Italics in the original.) See Julius A. Roth, "Some Contingencies of the Moral Evaluation and Control of Clientele: The Case of the Hospital Emergency Service," *American Journal of Sociology* 77 (March 1972): 839–856.

3. Judith Lorber describes how hospital staffs divide their patients into "problem" and "no problem" categories on the basis of interference with routines. See "Good Patients and Problem Patients: Conformity and Deviance in a General Hospital," *Journal of Health and Social Behavior* 16 (June 1975): 213–225.

4. Thomas S. Szasz and Marc H. Hollender, "The Basic Models of the Doctor-Patient Relationship," *Archives in Internal Medicine* 97 (1956): 585–592. The many ambulance patients who are unconscious or semiconscious, and thus require relationships that fit an alternative ("activity-passivity") model, are likely to be in the category of emergency runs and thus not evaluated as good or bad patients.

5. Betty Scalice, "Abuse of EMS: Is There a Remedy?" *Emergency* 10, no. 8 (August 1978): 51–56.

6. See Keith Griffiths, "A New Approach to System Abuse," *Paramedics International* 4, no. 3 (Fall 1979): 23–25.

7. A study of five hospitals by Roth found a range of 3 to 8 percent urgent cases, approximately 5 percent borderline, and the rest clearly not urgent. Julius A. Roth, "Utilization of the Hospital Emergency Department," *Journal of Health and Social Behavior* 12 (December 1971): 312–320. See also Geoffrey Gibson, O. W. Anderson, and G. Bugbee, *Emergency Medical Services in the Chicago Area*, Center for Health Administration Studies, University of Chicago, 1970.

8. Marvin A. Lavenhar, Robert S. Ratner, and E. Richard Weinerman, "Social Class and Medical Care: Indices of Nonurgency in Use of Hospital Emergency Services," *Medical Care* 6, no. 5 (September–October 1968).

9. In this judgment the attendants are distinguishing between legitimate and illegitimate patients in the same manner as the emergency department staffs studied by Roth ("Some Contingencies). For a review of the variety of biases demonstrated by practitioners in judging patients, see Solomon Papper, "The Undesirable Patient," *Journal of Chronic Diseases* 22 (1970): 777-779.

10. John T. Riley, Jr., "Riley's Rules for EMS," *Emergency* 12, no. 5 (May 1980): 83.

11. Kate Boyd, "The Public Inebriate: A Complex Problem," *JEMS: A Journal of Emergency Medical Services* 5, no. 2 (April 1980): 21-26.

12. See the account of "flooding out" or "breaking frame"—where the flow of emotion overcomes the formal demeanor of the social role—in Erving Goffman, *Encounters: Two Studies in the Sociology of Interaction* (Indianapolis: Bobbs-Merrill, 1961), pp. 55-61.

13. This condition is referred to by some physicians as "post traumatic stress disorder—chronic." It shows up in the form of flashbacks which are not mere recollections of an event, but an actual living out of the event as though the person were back in the traumatic situation.

14. Media campaigns in Dallas produced different results, in one case an increase in calls and in another a decrease. Ray F. Reed, "Job Satisfaction Survey of EMS Personnel," *The EMT Journal* 5, no. 1 (February 1981): 22. Reed also reports (p. 25) that a city council charge for any "no transport" calls reduced the number of unnecessary runs for about five months; in his opinion the publicity surrounding the voting of the charge was more effective than the financial penalty itself.

15. W. H. Lamm, "Dispatchers: Getting the Message Straight," *Emergency* 12, no. 6 (June 1980): 52-57.

16. In one case a 911 operator in Miami underestimated the calm report of a break-in in progress telephoned by a juvenile girl, who was discovered a few hours later to have been the victim of rape and murder. The dispatcher was demoted and disciplined. In Jacksonville a patient died during the delay while an ambulance dispatcher asked for more information. This dispatcher was also disciplined. See "Dispatcher Error May Have Contributed to Death," *JEMS: A Journal of Emergency Medical Services* 5, no. 2 (April 1980): 8.

17. The newspaper (which is not identified here to maintain the anonymity of the company) headlined the original story, "Ambulance Turned Down a Very Sick Man," and eventually followed it with an editorial asking, "How Careful Is Emergency Care?"

18. In Metropolis, when the paramedics have been instructed by their base physician to cease resuscitation efforts, they will call the privates to transport the body to a hospital to be pronounced. Although the attendants are safe in treating the body so, it is possibly not dead in a technical legal sense. In some cases "any competent person" may pronounce a body dead, but the criteria of competence are vague, and the pronouncer must still satisfy the person who signs the death certificate.

19. One of the most widely used EMT texts uses this general standard. See The Committee on Allied Health, American Academy of Orthopaedic Surgeons, *Emergency Care and Transportation of The Sick and Injured*, 2nd ed., revised (Chicago: American Academy of Orthopaedic Surgeons, 1977), pp. 82-83. The stan-

dard is not precise, because certain conditions, for example, cooler temperatures, can slow body processes and the brain's need for oxygen and extend the arrested patient's survival time beyond six minutes. Victims of exposure and cold water drowning should not be written off quickly. Emergency physicians say, "No one is dead until he is warm and dead."

20. See David Sudnow, "Dead on Arrival," *Transaction* 5, no. 1, excerpted from his book *Passing On: The Social Organization of Dying* (Englewood Cliffs, N.J.: Prentice-Hall, 1967), pp. 100-109. Douglas describes a number of variables that seem to influence the action taken by the ambulance crews. Dorothy Jean Douglas, *Occupational and Therapeutic Contingencies of Ambulance Services in Metropolitan Areas* (Ann Arbor, Michigan: University Microfilms, 1970), pp. 234-279.

21. The Committee on Allied Health, *Emergency Care*, p. 83.

22. In the opinion of a lawyer-paramedic, ". . . an EMT is not qualified to make the medical or clinical judgments or ethical decisions that death would be more humane or that the patient is or is not salvable. . . . The failure to resuscitate an otherwise viable patient can never be reversed nor can it be satisfactorily explained. There is no margin for error." *JEMS: A Journal of Emergency Medical Services* 6, no. 1 (January 1981): 41.

23. EMTs do not get much instruction on how to use their bodies effectively and safely in lifting, but many of them are aware of the potential for injury and informally advise each other. For one of the few discussions, see Thom Dick's article, "Look Out Behind You! Protecting Your Back," *JEMS: A Journal of Emergency Medical Services* 5, no. 10 (December 1980): 20-27.

24. The placebo, which is a pharmacologically inert substance or a treatment with no direct bearing on the medical problem, seems to have a potent symbolic value. Evidently the patient's belief that the treatment will be effective sometimes produces the desired effect. See Jerome Frank, "The Placebo Effect in Medical and Psychological Treatment," in his book *Persuasion and Healing* (Baltimore: The John Hopkins Press, 1961), pp. 65-74.

25. See R. Jack Ayres, Jr., "Patient Consent and the Law, Part 1: General Principles," *JEMS: A Journal of Emergency Medical Services* 5, no. 10 (December 1980) 33-35.

26. Ibid., "Part 2," p. 40.

27. Betty Scalice, "A Warning from Chicago," *JEMS: A Journal of Emergency Medical Services* 5, no. 10 (December 1980): 28-32.

28. James M. Henslin describes how cab drivers use stereotypes to minimize the danger from their fares in "What Makes for Trust?", in his book, *Down to Earth Sociology*, 3rd ed. (New York: The Free Press, 1981), pp. 90-102.

29. Douglas observed similar devices for self-protection in the ambulance companies she studied. *Occupational and Therapeutic Contingencies*, pp. 147-148.

30. Associated Press carried accounts of these incidents, datelined Chicago, on January 9 and January 16, 1981. The same routines are used elsewhere. A Baltimore firefighter assisting the paramedics said, "You get called up to the 11th floor of these projects and you're the only white person in the whole building. I don't care if they're bleeding to death, I'm not going up there until I call a (police) radio car to escort me up. I'm not putting my life in jeopardy for someone who may already be dead. I'll give it 100 percent, but I have to have some protection." Joe

Calderone, "Personnel Shortage Threatens Service," *Baltimore News American,* June 22, 1980, p. 7A. Police escort is tacitly considered essential in Boston and elsewhere. Betty Scalice, "Around the Nation," *JEMS: A Journal of Emergency Medical Services* 6, no. 2 (February 1981): 13.

31. In many situations the proper mode of address is unclear, for example, when one acquires a set of parents-in-law. A description of the difficulties of determining proper forms is given in Richard J. Gelles and Craig B. Little, "Forms of Address: Yardstick and Stumbling Block of Social Interaction," *Our Sociological Eye,* Arthur B. Shostak, ed. (Port Washington, N.Y.: Alfred Publishing Company, 1977), pp. 114-120.

32. Status differences can be seen when one role performer uses the familiar first name and the other uses the formal or polite form of address. The relationship between doctors and nurses is an example. See Erving Goffman, *Interaction Ritual* (Garden City, N.Y.: Doubleday, 1967), pp. 60-65.

33. The staff in the nursing home studied by Gubrium used a variety of forms of address for the patients, including first names (Mazie), last names with titles (Mr. Canfield), and slang names (honey). The uses seemed to vary with the patient's condition (alert or confused), the setting (staffing or ward), and the user (floor nurse or top staff). See Jaber F. Gubrium, *Living and Dying at Murray Manor* (New York: St. Martin's Press, 1975). Thelma Owens speaks for at least some older patients when she writes: "Another little courtesy I can dispense with is the habit some doctors have of calling me by my first name. . . . Young doctors seem especially eager to get on a first-name basis with old ladies. They are downright folksy as they tell their patient that her gall bladder must come out, but it's nothing that should bother a big girl like her. . . . But he can square everything by giving me my married name and my blood pressure reading and letting me go home." "Some Things to Decline in Your Declining Years," *Sunday Magazine, Metropolitan Daily,* April 5, 1981, p. 29.

34. See Gubrium on the designations "agitated," "disoriented," and "confused" in a nursing home. Gubrium, *Living and Dying at Murray Manor,* pp. 49-51.

35. Sudnow, "Dead on Arrival," p. 101.

36. As Rosenhan pointed out in connection with his investigation of psychiatric hospitals, ". . . elements are given meaning by the context in which they occur." Rosenhan found that the patient's behavior was interpreted to fit with his patient status. D. L. Rosenhan, "On Being Sane in Insane Places," *Science* 179 (January 19, 1973): 250-258. Ambulance patients are assessed in part on the basis of where they are picked up.

37. Andy Knott, in a series of articles on private ambulance services in Chicago, reported that the crews refer to patients from the public housing projects as "grunts." See "Let Him Die . . . ," *Chicago Tribune,* March 17, 1981, pp. 1, 8.

Notes for Chapter 7

1. One of the hobbyists in Metropolis was a health administrator who followed public service band dispatches closely enough to realize he was losing part of the

transmissions. He had not known that the ambulance crews switch to a secure frequency to talk with the hospitals. One couple claimed to have the scanner on all day and even to listen to it after they were in bed.

2. Comments from students, letters to newspaper editors, and other citizens reveal a great many misconceptions about sirens: that the volume can be adjusted by the crew, that they are intended to be used only for intersections, that they are prohibited by some jurisdictions and allowed by others, that if a siren is turned on or off in the middle of a block it is because the crew is going to lunch, that the siren is used to communicate with the hospital, and so on. Inevitably these comments convey a measure of hostility toward the ambulance services.

3. Reported on "Paul Harvey: The Rest of the Story," American Broadcasting Company Radio Network, June 30, 1980.

4. Associated Press and United Press International dispatches of November 6, 1979, reported this behavior at a game between Temple and Hawaii.

5. These three considerations parallel the rationale and some of the elements (perceived seriousness, perceived benefits, perceived barriers) of the Health Belief Model, which was formulated to explain the likelihood of one's taking (recommended preventative) health action. See M. H. Becker and L. A. Maiman, "Sociobehavioral Determinants of Compliance with Health and Medical Care Recommendations," *Medical Care* 13 (1975): 10-24.

6. See the representative articles on class and culture respectively by Earl Lomon Koos, "Illness in Regionville," pp. 9-14, and Mark Zborowski, "Cultural Components in Responses to Pain," pp. 118-133, in *Sociological Studies of Health and Illness,* Dorian Apple, ed. (New York: McGraw-Hill, 1960).

7. Roth anticipates that the number of people using the emergency department for routine medical care will increase as more people recognize its convenience in comparison with other forms of delivery. Julius A. Roth, "Utilization of the Hospital Emergency Department," *Journal of Health and Social Behavior* 12 (December 1971): 319.

8. Colman and Robboy point out that the geographic site of the incident, as well as the age of the patient and the time of day, affect whether a case will be defined as an emergency by witnesses. Clifford V. Colman and Howard Robboy, "The Social Construction of an Emergency," *Topics in Emergency Medicine* 1, no. 4 (January 1980): 61-66.

9. The bystander who intervenes in an emergency risks legal entanglements only if guilty of gross or wanton negligence that significantly departs from what a reasonable or prudent person might be expected to do under those circumstances. Many states have passed legislation to protect and thus encourage bystander intervention. See Betty Scalice, "The Good Samaritan Doctrine," *Emergency* 10, no. 10 (October 1978): 54-55.

10. George Moorhead provides a brief, wry, and accurate overview of the divergent interests and perspectives of related personnel in his article, "The EMS Jungle," *Emergency* 11, no. 4 (April 1979): 28-31.

11. We can refer to expectations that develop in the course of practice as "emergent roles," because they are not formally recognized, are more specific than traditional roles, and are in effect only in the presence of particular individuals.

12. Maya Angelou, *Gather Together in My Name* (New York: Random House, 1974), pp. 124-125.

13. Dorothy Jean Douglas, *Occupational and Therapeutic Contingencies of Ambulance Services in Metropolitan Areas* (Ann Arbor, Michigan: University Microfilms, 1970), p. 70.

14. Lawrence Hatfield thinks the relative of the patient may be the biggest management problem the EMT faces. "Controlling the Trauma Scene," *The EMT Journal* 4, no. 4 (December 1980): 29-31.

15. This term is used by William R. Roush, "Management of the Emergency Scene," *The EMT Journal* 4, no. 3 (September 1980): 27-28. He refers to J. E. George, "Medical Intervenors," *The EMT Legal Bulletin* 4 (1978): 1-6.

16. James O. Page, "Beechwood Revisited," *Paramedics International*, March-April 1978: 20-23.

17. "Paramedics report that they experience their greatest difficulty when they encounter well-meaning physicians at the scene of an emergency or are called to a physician's office to render aid." Fire Captain/Paramedic Gary P. Morris offers some suggestions on how to deal with these difficulties in "Thank You, Doctor, But Please Stand Back," *JEMS: A Journal of Emergency Medical Services* 5, no. 2 (April 1980): 35-36.

18. A story that circulated among EMTs gives an idea of their estimates of the skills of untrained law enforcement personnel: "At an accident scene a deputy asked what he could do to help. An EMT, earnestly working on a bleeder, snapped out, 'Get me some four-by-fours [sterile bandages].' The deputy looked around, then asked, 'Where the hell are you going to find sawn lumber around here? Would some planks do?' "

19. The lack of EMT status does not mean the police are therefore ineffective in dealing with medical emergencies. Most police have had first aid instruction, and some of them employ it well. For example, one regular California Highway Patrol officer has delivered seven babies on duty during a fifteen-year career (Associated Press, August 23, 1980), and a police dispatcher in Michigan saved the life of a stroke victim who could not speak on the phone by getting him to communicate with a series of taps (Associated Press, February 8, 1981).

20. Even though the two services have different priorities on the scene, their relationship can be cordial and effective if they take the time to recognize their differences and compromise. See Robert Ciupa, "Death, Police, and Casualty Care," *JEMS: A Journal of Emergency Medical Services* 5, no. 6 (August 1980): 39-41.

21. Julius A. Roth, "The Neccessity and Control of Hospitalization," *Social Science and Medicine* 6 (1972): 111-119.

22. B.Z. gave the commissioner of health another example of the lack of coordination among the units: "We were sent to an automobile accident. Squad 18 was there, but it was an extrication [of the patient from the wreckage] and they didn't know what to do. The woman had a little neurological deficit so we shortboarded her. We had the collar and the Kling in place and were setting the straps when Mobile 2 arrived. We didn't even know they had been called. The paramedics pushed us aside, tore off the straps and Kling and removed the shortboard. They extricated the patient by hand and put her on a longboard lying on the cot. I heard someone at the hospital say she arrived a quadriplegic."

23. The technically sophisticated are so fascinated with their techniques that they sometimes lose sight of their primary purpose. When this happens in ambu-

lance work, EMTs have reason to complain that it has progressed from the merely-transportation evil of "swoop and scoop" to the IV-therapy-first evil of "grab and stab." In both cases basic life support practices are overlooked. For an example of this problem, see the readers' letters in "Bad Air in NYC," *Emergency* 13, no. 1 (January 1981): 5.

24. The privates complain about nursing homes delaying too long before transferring patients to a hospital, thus forcing the ambulances to run hot. A nurse at one of the homes said the problem is that they always have difficulty contacting the patient's physician to get authorization for the transfer.

25. This term is used in the Baltimore system. Joe Calderone, "Paramedics: On the Street, It's Different," *Baltimore News American*, June 24, 1980, p. 1A.

26. A story covering the incidence of these bans was carried in one of the Metropolis newspapers on October 24, 1980.

27. Robert K. McCullough, "Burning Out," *The EMT Newsletter*, no. 8 (November 1980): 4.

28. Gail Walraven, "Face to Face," Part I, *Emergency* 11, no. 4 (April 1979): 47.

29. Just one reference among many is Robert Elling, 'Stress as Related to the EMT-P," *The EMT Journal* 4, no. 4 (December 1980): 34.

30. Douglas claimed that for the cases she studied hospital staff "realize the men need certain non-standard items of equipment and welcome their taking the initiative in 'lifting' whatever first-aid materials they think they need." *Occupational and Therapeutic Contingencies*, p. 221 (note 39).

31. Gail Walraven, "Face to Face," Part II, *Emergency* 11, no. 5 (May 1979): 63.

32. Knowledge and coordination are both problems, according to current research. A study of Los Angeles hospitals conducted by the *Long Beach Independent Press-Telegram* found that of 63 sample emergency department cases resulting in death, 7 (11 percent) of the deaths were "clearly preventable," 30 (48 percent) were "possibly preventable," and 26 (41 percent) were "not preventable." This level of treatment was explained as being due to inadequately trained staff, lack of medical specialists, misdiagnoses, and slow handling. The patient is therefore not necessarily safe, even if he survives the prehospital phase of EMS, and the EMTs' estimation of the insufficiencies of EDs may have a basis in fact. United Press International dispatch, December 29, 1980, datelined Los Angeles.

33. These experiences are not peculiar to Liberty or to Metropolis. See the introduction to Walraven, "Face to Face," Part I, p. 47.

34. Ibid., Part II, p. 63.

35. Ibid, Part I, p. 49.

36. Other services make similar complaints. A Baltimore paramedic was reported as saying, "You're looking for a kind word sometimes from these hospital people, like 'Hey, you did a good job on that one.' Instead, they say 'Why didn't you do this, and why didn't you do that?' They work in a sterile hospital atmosphere and for them, it all goes smoothly. They don't know what it's like on the street. They don't have the family beating on your back, yelling for you to 'do something, do something, don't let him die.' When you've got people screaming at

you, I don't care who you are, you get rattled." Calderone, "Paramedics: On the Street, It's Different," p. 4A.

37. David Allan et al., "Learning to Work Together," *Emergency* 11, no. 6 (June 1979): 60-62.

Notes for Chapter 8

1. Much of this information is based on *Status Report: Emergency Medical Services in Metropolitan County,* a mimeographed statement prepared and circulated by the Emergency Government Office of Metropolitan County in the fall of 1975.

2. The state's population estimates for 1978 put Metropolitan County at about 961,000 and the city of Metropolis at about 618,000. "Close-in Suburbs Join City in Population Loss," *Metropolitan Daily,* August 11, 1978, Part I, p. 1.

3. This idea is explored in Donald L. Metz, "Emergency Medical Service Systems: A Case of Structural Lag," mimeo., Department of Sociology, Anthropology, and Social Work, Marquette University, Milwaukee, Wisconsin, 1978.

4. See William F. Ogburn, *On Culture and Social Change* (Chicago: University of Chicago Press, 1964), p. 86.

5. "Annual Health Care Plan Underway," *ECHSA Outlook* 4, no. 7 (August/September 1980): 1. By the end of 1980 eighty-four communities in the state had adopted the 911 emergency telephone system.

6. Resistance to establishing a single emergency telephone number has been found elsewhere. See, for example, J.H.U. Brown and the Southwest Research Consortium, *The Politics of Health Care* (Cambridge, Mass.: Ballinger, 1978), p. 122.

7. These claims were made by the medical directors of the paramedic program. Metropolis's success rate of 41.5 percent in resuscitating patients in ventricular fibrillation was compared with reports from studies that put Seattle's rate at 38.7 percent and Miami's at 33.6 percent. "Area Paramedics Rate High in Saving Lives," *Metropolitan Daily,* March 18, 1979, Part II, p. 1. In 1980 the program claimed a success rate of 45.6 percent. "In My Opinion: Paramedic Program Still Has a Long Way to Go," *Metropolitan Daily,* April 10, 1981, Part, I, p. 14.

8. "A Day in the Life of Metropolis," *Metropolitan Daily,* August 17, 1978, Part II, p. 1.

9. "If the City Budget Were Cut 20%," *Metropolitan Daily,* September 6, 1978, Part II, p. 1.

10. "City's Paramedic Service Suffering from Attrition," *News of Metropolis,* May 16, 1981, Part I, p. 5.

11. Ibid.

12. The city's Legislative Reference Bureau reported to the council that ambulance costs had increased 141 percent from 1967 to 1979. It estimated that, given the $75 fee in place when the system began, to keep up with costs, the privates should have been charging $81.15 in late 1978 and $90.73 in late 1979, rather than the $75 they had been receiving through that period. "Ambulance Firms Seek Higher Rate," *Metropolitan Daily,* July 27, 1980, Part II, p. 1.

13. "Ambulance Fee May Not Change," *Metropolitan Daily,* October 18, 1978, Part II, p. 1.

14. "Ambulance Firms Seek Higher Rate."

15. Newspapers rarely present the viewpoint of the ambulance workers in the field. Stories are much more likely to give the perspectives of complaining citizens and patients or of functionaires of higher status—government officials, physicians, members of advisory boards. As a result, politicians do not learn much about EMS from newspaper accounts. Thus, when a story does touch on field operations, there is a good chance it will get a somewhat surprised reaction from the authorities.

16. "Probe of Ambulance Use Sought," *Metropolitan Daily,* June 5, 1980, Part II, p. 15.

17. "Why the Orange Strip?" *The EMT Newsletter* 6 (August 1980): 7.

18. "President's Message," *EMTA Journal,* November-December 1979: 3.

19. See particularly Chapter V, "Implications for Further Study and Conclusion," in Dorothy Jean Douglas, *Occupational and Therapeutic Contingencies of Ambulance Services in Metropolitan Areas* (Ann Arbor, Michigan: University Microfilms, 1970), pp. 298-309.

20. For two accounts of the contribution of emergency medical workers (both prehospital and in the emergency department), see Nick Arnett, "Who Saved Mr. Reagan?" *Emergency* 13 (May 1981): 58-59; and Jim Malone, "Washington Report," *JEMS: A Journal of Emergency Medical Services* 6, no. 5 (May 1981): 17-18.

21. The event occurred and was reported by local television stations on September 10, 1980.

22. Jan Schwettman, "Nuggets," *JEMS: A Journal of Emergency Medical Services* 6, no. 1 (January 1981): 12.

23. (Chicago, Illinois: American Academy of Orthopaedic Surgeons, 1977), pp. 89-93.

24. Some examples of relevant articles are: Henry J. Heimlich, "Errors in Standards?" *Emergency* 13, no. 3 (March 1981): 22-23; Henry J. Heimlich, "Back Blows Are Death Blows," *Emergency Medical Services* 8 (1979): 88; E. L. Nagel et al., "The Heimlich Maneuver Versus Back Blows for Choking Victims," *Emergency Medical Services* 9 (1980): 11-38; Edward A. Patrick, "Choking: A Questionnaire to Find the Most Effective Treatment," *Emergency* 12, no. 7 (July 1980): 59-64; Joseph S. Redding, "The Choking Controversy: Critique of Evidence on the Heimlich Maneuver," *EMTA Journal* (November-December 1980): 5-8.

25. See, for example, "Letters," *Emergency* 13, no. 5 (May 1981): 6.

26. "MAST Device: May We?" *The EMT Newsletter,* June 1980: 3.

Notes for Chapter 9

1. "3 Life Stories: Why More Survive 'Sudden Death,' " *Metropolitan Daily,* May 31, 1981, Part II, p. 1.

2. See the account of a Seattle hospital's admissions and policy committee in Renée C. Fox and Judith Swazey, *The Courage to Fail* (Chicago: University of Chicago Press, 1974).

3. Rick Carlson, *The End of Medicine* (New York: John Wiley and Sons, 1976), p. 126.

4. Reported in "Inside EMS," *JEMS: A Journal of Emergency Medical Services* 5, no. 10 (December 1980): 7, 10.

5. Associated Press dispatch of April 7, 1981, datelined Washington, D.C.

6. This perspective parallels the view of blood donations expressed by Richard M. Titmuss in *The Gift Relationship: From Human Blood to Social Policy* (New York: Random House, 1972). The perspective is explored more fully in Donald L. Metz, "The Emergency Medical Services Volunteer: Expression of Social Solidarity," mimeo., Department of Sociology, Anthropology, and Social Work, Marquette University, Milwaukee, 1980.

7. See the reference to Elling in note 38 of Chapter 5.

8. This is based on a comment attributed to Rocco Morando, National Registry executive director, by Jan Schwettman, "Nuggets," *JEMS: A Journal of Emergency Medical Services* 5, no. 5 (July 1980): 12.

appendix a

Participant Observation of an Ambulance Crew

This project grew out of my interest in medical sociology. I wanted to take a look from inside the medical care system to get a more complete picture of how it operates. Training as an EMT seemed a very economical way to accomplish that purpose. (However, one of my discoveries was that ambulance workers are in many ways on the outside too.) In the EMT classes it was easy to do sociology. The trainees were a diverse lot. It was natural to ask questions or just listen during coffee breaks, and note-taking was a legitimate classroom activity. Several years later, as an employee at Liberty, I could not blend into the crowd as readily.

On an Ambulance Crew

When I was ready to work I called three or four ambulance companies listed in the yellow pages. I visited two of them. Liberty's quarters were shabby, but the personnel seemed pleasant. Pete, one of the owners, said they were adding only qualified EMTs to the roster. He had no objections to my doing research, but he was not willing to ask the state officials to allow me to take the EMT examination until I had made a few runs and was sure I wanted to do this kind of work. The owner of the second company also accepted my plan to do research. Moreover, he signed a letter to the state and thus got the examining process underway. In spite of the second company's ready cooperation, or perhaps because it seemed too casual, I felt more comfortable with Liberty and did my work with them.

The workers at Liberty were friendly and eager to talk about the job. But for a while they had difficulty placing me as a person. The bare spot on the top of my head and the gray in my beard clearly indicated that I was a generation older than most of them. They knew I couldn't be earning a living there, since the pay was so low and I was working fewer hours than they were. They entertained the idea that I was a siren freak looking for cheap thrills. I told them I was a sociology teacher from the university doing research on ambulances. They interpreted this to mean either that I was a part-time lecturer or that I worked at the two-year technical college. They translated my remarks about research to mean that I was writing a book, and throughout my tour there were people who continued to imagine they would appear in a novel. My position was just as ambiguous from the other side; long time associates and neighbors assumed I was simply observing on ambulances rather than actually doing the work.

Eventually a reasonably accurate story explaining my presence began to circulate. The Liberty people joked about "Dr. Metz" on the crew. One of the fire fighters, the irrepressible Palermo, who wanted to be written about, referred to me as the "the professor." Both hospital and fire personnel would give mock warnings when I was around that they were being watched. Lyle brought me some sociologically oriented articles from EMT publications.

Most of the time I kept a low profile. The slow periods at the company provided opportunities to make notes or to talk. I accepted the role of novice and asked questions of my more experienced colleagues. I tried not to pry into personal matters and I avoided expressing strong opinions or passing on gossip. Whenever I could I offered the "immediate reciprocities" [John Lofland, *Analyzing Social Settings* (Belmont, Calif.: Wadsworth, 1971), p. 98] that are necessary contributions to the informal social network. I would listen, converse, sympathize, and occasionally advise. I would buy meals and snacks for my partners now and then. And I washed the dishes and emptied the ashtrays in quarters often enough that it became a routine. Jase pointed out, "Tanner can never find an ashtray because Don's always washing them."

My EMT skills were not exceptional. I depended on my crew chiefs. My bedside manner was acceptable and my paperwork was neat, but I missed a lot of blood pressures. I contributed to the well-being of several patients but was unable to stave off death for one. The biggest recognition of my service was a compliment from one of the emergency department nurses (delivered by Louie) on my radio report during a run to the hospital.

The crews apparently were interested in how I would adjust to the setting. Eventually I understood that they were looking for evidence that I was being influenced, that they were socializing me. They were delighted when I began to swear. They warmed up noticeably after I resorted to throwing incomplete reports and trip slips on the floor of the ambulance cab during a busy shift.

Gradually I found a place in the company. I joined the others in being the butt of jokes. Flash felt secure enough to wise-crack about how I lost one of Liberty's customers the night a patient died in the rig while I was doing CPR. I liked all the Liberty people, though I felt more comfortable with some than with others. I am not aware of having been considered anyone's enemy. After I had stopped regular work and returned to teaching at the university, Tanner said he told the others to blow the siren when they went past my building so I would get homesick and work a few more shifts.

However cordial our relationships, I was never one of the gang. There was an age gap, and it did no good to pretend it wasn't there. Lyle told me he sometimes found it awkward to act as crew chief when I was obviously senior in age and education. This awkwardness was caused partly by outsiders turning to me as the probable leader of the crew. There were also cultural differences. I was teased about using strange expressions (like calling a corpse's throat a tunnel of decay) and uncommon words (like "opt" instead of "choose," though Jilly pointed out that Jase was always "opting" for something). On occasion academic jargon would slip out, as when I mentioned that my neighborhood was mixed because there were a lot of working class people there. ("Wait a minute! What is this working class shit? I thought you meant it was racially integrated. What the hell are we?") The clearest indicator that I remained in a category apart was that the other EMTs never called me "fucker," a common expression of companionship.

I am grateful that, in spite of the differences between us, the other EMTs were willing to accept me and even to trust me. I was not aware that they attempted to cover up any of their activities (from their private pornography collections to the five finger discount). I think the main reason for this was that they did not feel they had anything to hide. Also, they seemed to read me as not threatening. At any rate, I found no evidence that the workers promoted a front to keep me at a distance from the reality of the setting. I am satisfied that I had access to what I needed to see. If I failed to notice important things, the fault was mine.

Participant Observation

There were many times when being a participant on the ambulance got in the way of my observing. The demands of the moment when running hot or on the scene prevent the EMT from casually scanning his surroundings or reflecting on the behavior he sees. Because his actions are being judged by others involved in the ongoing activity, the participant's emotions are brought into play and influence his judgment. Moreover, the fact that the patient's well-being is at stake necessarily distracts all but the most callous participants from their less immediate goals. At the same time, my attempts to be an observer sometimes prevented my improving my skills as a participant. I was too interested in the broader picture to concentrate on certain details. I never learned the street locations well enough to drive hot; I never mastered the exact quantities of supplies that were supposed to be in the rigs; I never learned all the ten-signals or any of the combinations for raising the hospitals on the encoders.

For some research, observers can do sociological field work better than participants can. The outsider can enumerate and analyze observable behaviors without the distraction of having constantly to respond to others. However, the observer's judgments may be accurate only for those behaviors within his empathetic repertoire. When the acts and actors are clearly different from the observer's familiar world, then participation in the setting being studied can prevent some otherwise tempting distortions. There are many aspects of ambulance work I would not have understood or even known about had I not been a participant.

This is not to say that participants and observers necessarily draw different conclusions because of their different perspectives. Reading Dorothy Douglas's dissertation on ambulance work was enormously reassuring for me. Although she was trained as a nurse and rode ambulances as an observer, her experiences were strikingly similar to my own. It convinced me that we were indeed talking about a similar reality and that the conditions of the work produced similar behaviors in different places. At the same time, there were significant differences in our accounts, some of which can be linked to the character of our involvement in the settings.

First, Douglas seemed to be somewhat less sympathetic toward ambulance workers than I have been. This can be explained in part by the general improvement in emergency medical services over the ten years that separated our studies. However, Douglas approached the ambulance study as a nurse and an outsider, and both of these roles distanced her from her subjects. She had no particular reason to give the workers the benefit of the doubt. As an EMT, however, I identified to some extent with the people I was studying. Since I was only temporarily an EMT, the identification was not complete, but it was probably sufficient to incline me to a somewhat more favorable view of their activities. Either approach carries the certainty of some distortion, but they work in opposite directions.

Second, the demands of any job (the confusion, the boredom, the aches of an unnatural posture) may be impossible to understand fully unless one tries to meet them. Filling out an EMT report seems simple enough until you undertake it on the run. Getting the main points of a patient's history couldn't be easier until the distractions of the scene interrupt and deflect the flow of information. How can the observer know that failure to get a complete set of vitals is not always a matter of laziness or inattention? Because of her medical training and her close association with ambulance personnel, Douglas may have appreciated more than other observers the difficulties of the job. Even so, she was occasionally inclined to attribute work insufficiencies to the character of the workers. Put another way, participation may erode somewhat the observer's idealized standards of what should be taking place.

Third, participation helps the researcher to recognize the feelings that accompany certain kinds of behavior. The participant understands fatigue after a busy shift, depression after losing a patient, irritation with unco-operative bystanders, worry about a dead-end career, frustration at con-flicting orders or interpretations. The observer might find these matters comprehensible but ambiguous, or might be predisposed to dismiss the ac-tors as unreasonable. In short, the participant might share with the workers an anxiety that cannot be appreciated by the observer who does not participate. Douglas was very sensitive to both the workers' feelings and her own contribution to stimulating those feelings.

Fourth, participation usually requires going through a training program that socializes the worker into a specific set of meanings. These meanings are essential to an understanding of the worker's perspective. Attitudes to-ward physicians, nurses, and other EMS workers are outlined during the formal training period; they are filled in during on-the-job experiences. Douglas found that her subjects had had little formal training. Thus, she was able to be present during much of the socialization of the newer atten-dants. A decade later the education of EMTs and RNs is sufficiently differ-ent with regard to emergency services that participation in attendant train-ing would be advantageous for a nurse-researcher.

The biggest differences between my report and that of Douglas, how-ever, are due not to research style but to the passage of time. Douglas did have problems getting behind the fronts the ambulance services put up to deceive her, while I was able to move quietly behind facades, because as a participant, I had access to unconcealable events. But Douglas's discover-ies differed from my own most sharply in matters related to the training, background, equipment, and techniques of the attendants. In the decade between her research and mine, private ambulance operations have changed from a loosely regulated cartage business to a formally recognized occupational category with specific requirements for personnel, materials, and procedures. The similarities in our two accounts suggest that custom and social structure are important determinants of ambulance work; the differences show the importance of political action and government policy in causing social change, and offer hope for even greater improvements in the future.

appendix b
Types of Ambulance Assignments

My best estimate of the time devoted to different activities by ambulance workers is based on a log of the assignments I had during part of my service with Liberty. This log is not necessarily a representative sample of the company's work pattern. It only covers a period from late spring through early autumn. Nor does it include data from the "first shift" (midnight to 8:00 AM), when there is usually less action and a lower average number of assignments than is true for the other shifts. These biases suggest that the log may slightly overestimate crew activity. I am not aware of other systematic distortions in the log.

The log covers 541 hours of duty time, during which my crew received 337 assignments. I use the term assignment to refer to an instance of an ambulance being sent out of quarters by the dispatcher for company business. It does not include routine maintenance of the vehicles (like getting gas), which the personnel take care of between runs, nor does it include personal business of the EMTs (like eating or cashing a check). On the average, there was one assignment every hour and thirty-six minutes, or about two every three hours. However, the workload was not evenly distributed. During eight-hour periods, there were as few as two assignments (on three occasions) and as many as eleven (on two occasions). Once my crew spent eight boring hours at a garage waiting for the repair of a rig, and another time we spent eight hours in the rain at the Riverside Arts Festival; on neither occasion did we make a single run.

The frequency of different kinds of ambulance assignments is shown in Table B-1. About 16 percent of the assignments were preparations for runs that did not occur (stand-by or head-to) or errands (picking up lunch for the owner, for example, or getting company mail from the post office). These were almost always carried out when business was slow and there were several crews in quarters. Since another 6 percent of the assignments were hot runs that did not result in patient contact, nearly one-fourth of the

Table B-1

DISTRIBUTION OF AMBULANCE ASSIGNMENTS

Type of Assignment	Frequency
Assignments other than runs:	
Errand	14
Stand-by (recalled without run)	11
Head-to (recalled without run)	28
Hot runs without patient contact:	
Cancelled en route	17
False alarm	2
Runs with patient contact but no transport:	
Back up another crew	2
No transport:	
No medical need	13
Refused transport	11
Transported by others	6
Runs involving patient transport:	
Scheduled run	47
Emergency run:	
Good run	40
Routine run	58
Shit call	88
Total	337

crew activities required no emergency medical skills. For an additional 10 percent of the assignments, the responding crew did make contact but did not have primary responsibility for the patient.

The remaining assignments, almost 70 percent of the total, involved patient transports. The largest proportion of these (about 25 percent of the total number of assignments) were what the crews called "shit calls" —apparent misuse of the ambulance. Routine emergency runs and scheduled runs together accounted for nearly half of the transports. The cases that had some element of a genuine emergency, those the crews called "good runs," occurred not quite once in eight assignments, according to my interpretation. A more experienced EMT for whom most of the work had become routine would consider good runs to be even less frequent than that.

Table B-2

DISTRIBUTION OF LOG PATIENTS' AGE BY GENDER

Age	Females(%)	Males(%)
Under 21	13	25
21-40	25	23
41-60	22	33
61-80	26	12
Over 80	14	8
Total Percent	100	101*
Total Number	137	128

*Percentages do not total 100 because of rounding.

The total numbers of men and women among the patients contacted were nearly equal, but the proportions varied by age group. The age and gender distribution is shown in Table B-2. The median age of female patients was 50 years and of males 43 years, almost certainly reflecting the greater longevity of the females. Men patients predominated throughout the under-20 category—among children, teenagers, and postadolescents. The genders were equally represented in the marriage and child-bearing years. In late middle age the majority of the patients were again men, but after age 60 most were female.

Slightly more than three-fourths of the patients contacted were white. A few of these spoke a language other than English. Some 15 percent of the patients were black, and another 8 percent might be classified as nonwhite. The white crews had difficulty understanding (not always because of language) some of the black patients and all of the Spanish speakers.

The runs required the use of at least twenty-six different items of equipment, not including cot coverings (sheets, pillowcases, absorbent pads, and towels). The items used most often on the logged runs, in order of frequency, were bandages, oxygen, orthopedic stretcher, cold packs, backboards, IV pole, and leg or arm splints. Some runs that did not call for equipment did require special positioning (shock, side) or monitoring (keep awake). The crews were likely to consider calls that involved equipment or specific procedures good runs.

Nearly all the patients were delivered to hospitals. Just over 5 percent were taken to their homes or to nursing homes. The logged patients were taken to seventeen different hospitals, though 59 percent of the transports were to four hospitals in different sectors of the city. These hospitals were considered appropriate for general emergency services. Patients with specific technical needs (burns, major trauma, childhood disease) might be taken to other hospitals. When the crews were suspicious about the patient's medical problem, they would go to the most convenient facility. In the case of drunks, they would try to drop the patient at an emergency room where the staff's displeasure would not cause problems for the crews later.

index